What is Bi Polar Disorder?

Putting the Pieces Together

Table of Contents

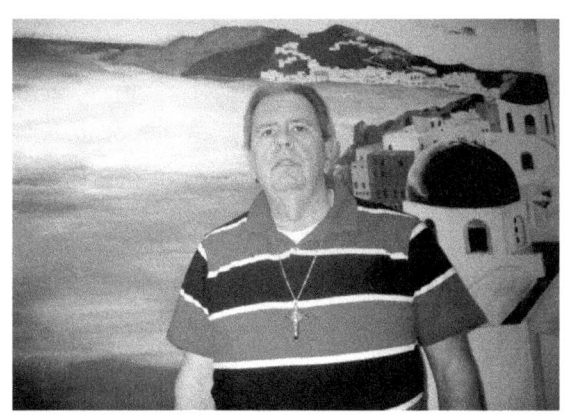

Revised July 2017

4th Edition
Published by BDS Distributors
Copyright 2014 by BDS Distributors

Chapter 1

Introduction

Hello, let me introduce myself. My name is Bruce D. Smith. I do not know where to begin my story. My father was a very good provider for our family. I can remember when I was very young like five or six years old both of my parents smoked cigarettes. My mother, one winter came down with a very bad case of bronchitis. It was so bad that she could not smoke. This was the best thing that happened to her because she stopped smoking. My father, on the other hand continue to smoke until the time of his death, January 17, 1988.

My sister and I always had a very good Christmas. My father would put a certain amount of money aside for us for Christmas presents. He would start his shopping in September and be done by Thanksgiving.

Sometimes we would go to church on Christmas Eve. I have always enjoyed the Christmas season. I could remember looking forward to Christmas and Easter vacation when I was in school.

I consider myself to be a C average student. If I only had applied myself my average could have been higher. But you know as the saying goes you cannot go back to the, "What if's." I have been going to college and all of my classes except for math I get A's and B's. I do apply myself to all of my classes now and I can see the difference.

Chapter 2

The Beginning of
My Mental Illness

My mental illness started way before I knew anything about mental illness. Therefore, I thought it was just normal for the things I would do.

Let me start from the beginning when I was about five years old. My sister had to have her tonsils out. My parents gave her a gift for being sick. She was in the hospital for a few days. Well I had the old fashion GI Joe doll. I liked the Marine Uniform they had for him at that time. So, I thought I could do the same thing as my sister did. I acted as having a sore throat. This was how my sisters' illness started. So, my father took me to the doctor. Well the doctor was on to me. He told my father that I did not have tonsillitis I had schoolitis. Needless to say, I did not get the GI Joe doll uniform which I wanted.

My illness did not stop there. It continued to Junior high school. I did not seem to have fit in at school when I was in the eighth grade. It

was time for me to go onto high school and I had more friends in the seventh grade then I did in my own grade. I did not want to move onto high school I wanted to just stay at junior high and stay back. So, what I did on purpose I started to fail in my subjects. Well my guidance counselor caught wind of this and he had a meeting with my mother and me. I got into a big argument with them both in the meeting. After the meeting, they convinced me into doing better in my classes so I can move on to high school.

I felt as though I would have to have people I like to feel sorry for me to get their attention. I liked this one girl, she was a freshman and I was a sophomore. So, I thought I would have to do something to get her attention. At the time, I was working at a doctor's office. Back in those days there was no problem with aids, infections, or drug use. They did not lock up needles and ones which were used just got thrown in the garbage. I would take the ones out of the garbage and take them home with me. I would get a pimple and I would inject some liquid soap into the needle then inject my pimple with it. This would cause an infection

eventually. The infection sometimes would get so bad I would have to go to the family surgeon to have it lanced. I would have to put a big patch on it and sometimes it would cause my eye to close. I thought this was so cool at the time and I would get the students, especially the girl I liked to feel sorry for me. This went on for a couple of years till I realized this did nothing at all. I even went as far as injecting my leg with this many time. It puzzled my doctors. They wondered why the infection would keep coming back from time to time. Eventually the surgeon cut out part of the skin around the infection. Boy was I in pain when the infections got bad. Finally, I got tired of the pain and realized this was getting me nowhere so I stopped doing it. I am paying for it till this day. The area the doctor cut the skin around the infection is all numb. If I stand long I get pain in the area. So, I guess you can say I am paying it in the long run.

Chapter 3

My Addictions

Well sad to say I turned 18 and I guess that was when I did all the things that I should not have done. That was when my life was to make a big change and would be a negative impact for the rest of my life. It was when I started to smoke cigarettes and to drink. One of my friends from time to time would offer me a cigarette and that was just the beginning of an ugly, nasty, and very addictive habit. Do not get me wrong I am not blaming my friend for this I am the only one to be the blame. I can remember what I liked the best out of smoking was when I lit up I would get a buzz, a short of a high off it. Every morning I would leave a half hour early to go to work so I could enjoy that first cigarette of the day. As time went on the more I smoked and then the more my health went downhill. I had trouble with my lungs when I was a baby. I had pneumonia when I was six months old. Then to top it off just before I started to smoke January 1978, I was in the hospital for pneumonia. After I stared to smoke I would get sick with bronchitis a lot. Boy did my life make a turn to the worse when that magic age came around. I would go out to the bars on the weekends with my friends. I guess you could say back then I was working for the weekends. All the money I made I would spend on the weekends. We would go to the Go-Go bars and of course when I would drink the more I smoked. I did not realize however; I was becoming addicted to one of the worst habits that anyone can do. After a while I did not care about anything but my cigarettes and drinking. I knew my health was getting worse as time went by. I was gaining weight fast. I would get light headed a lot and felt dizzy from time to time especially when I would come down with bronchitis.

I got laid off from my job in 1983 for about six months. You would think because of money I would cut back on things but I did not it just got worse. I did collect unemployment but I did not care. I drank and smoked all of my money up. I was very fortunate because I still lived at

home with my parents.

Chapter 4

The Calm before the Storm

It is Christmas Eve December 1987. I am fighting a battle with bronchitis otherwise all is going good. My night is going to be a very busy and late one. Tonight, I go to my friend's houses to play Santa Claus for their children. I start off at 6pm and who knows what time it is going to end. This night it is going to be 1:30am. I make Bob and Joann's house to be the last one because I usually stay there for a while and visit. I love doing this, just to see the expression on the kid's faces when they think I do not know they are there. I remember this day as I am writing this right now as if it happened yesterday. Such a pleasant thought to bring back to my mind for those dark days which I have. I, like everyone else did not know what the following year was going to bring. Wow what a change it will be not only would the carpet underneath me be taken away but I was going to move to a total new state, climate, setting and so on.

Chapter 5

New York City
December
1987

My boss from work and his girlfriend invited me to go to New York

City with them during our vacation. So, I went with them despise my

health. He drove right over and parked on one of the side streets. There

was this chill in the air. It was the Christmas chill. I was not cold. It

was the type of chill that would warm you up when you were a kid all

dressed and went to play in the snow. It was a fond memory to bring

the Christmas Memories alive in us. However, things were soon to

change. We went to St. Patrick's Cathedral. I treated all of us to a

horse drawn carriage ride around the Cathedral.   Then we went over to

Rockefeller Center. What a beautiful site, the Christmas tree was all lit

up. I never saw this in person before. We walk through the areas where

the stores had their windows decorated and boy what a sight it was.

This was the first time I was over there like this. I really enjoyed it.

Thanks Jack and Rose. I did not forget.

Well as usual the holidays came and went. The good stuff usually does not stay with us long.

In the next few days we will celebrate the New Year. That was what I call my holiday. I always would get drunk on New Year Eve. Ah the next day would I regret what I did the night before. I would always have too much to drink and yes, I paid for it the next morning.

Thank God, many years to follow I succeed at stopping one of my worst addictions and that was drinking alcohol.

Chapter 6

The Warning

Now it is Friday, January 15, 1988. My friend Cathy wants to go and have her palm read. She asks me if I want to go with her. So, we both decide to go. This lady to me was on the level. There was another palm reader in town but she was a rip off. She took me for a ride one time for $400.00. The only reason I paid it was because I did not want to take any chances of having anything done to me. I guess you may say I was superstitious. This one we went to only ask for donations, whatever you want to give. There was no set price. She always has a long line of people waiting to see her. We got to her house and yes there is a long line waiting to go in to see her. She was so good that people wait on line for her. We were getting closer to be our turn to see the woman. Well I go in and sit down and she tells me about my grandfathers that one of them was going to die. I tell her I did not know them. They were both dead when I was born. Now she hits home. She says to me, "You father is going to die VERY soon." Boy this hit me for a little while but then I did not take it to heart. Cathy went in and she was very accurate also about what was going on in her life at the time.

Chapter 7

The Worst Day
Of
My Life

Sunday came and I was working the midnight shift. I have been working overtime this weekend so it was busy for me. I did not stop by my parent's house over. I had stuff to do during the day then I laid down in the afternoon to take a nap. My mother called me about 5:30pm. She was very upset. She said, "I cannot wake your father up for dinner." I told her to try again. She said she did. I told her to call the police and have the ambulance come and I will be on my way. I went out to the living room and told my roommate Ricky what was going on. Ricky said, "Ah you will get down there and he will be ok." I told him what happen to me when I went to the palm reader on Friday. I left right away. My parents lived about 30 minutes from me but it took me 20. I got on Route 80 and drove 80. Well ok maybe not exactly 80 but close to it. On my way, down all I could think of my father being ok. He would be sitting in his chair and yelling at my mother for calling the police and ambulance for nothing. This is all I can think of all the way down to their house. We do not always get what we want. I got down to their house and all I see was first aid vehicles blocking the road at their house. I just parked where ever I could. I ran into their house to see how he was. He was upstairs in his bed room. I went to go up their but one of the first aiders I knew came down the stairs and stopped me. I asked him how my father was. He said to me you father is very sick that I could not go up there yet. The paramedics were working on him. I went over to the phone and call Ricky up because I was expecting some phone calls. I told him what was going on. Then a guy I did not recognize came over to me. He had the paramedic emblem on his shirt so I decided to get off the phone. He wanted me to stay on the phone but I hung up too quickly. He asked me who I was. I told me I was his son. He said to me that they did what they could; however your father passed away. . Wow did it hit me. He asked where my mother was. I told him next door. The

paramedic asked me if I wanted him to go and tell her or if I wanted to.
I told him I would. I quit smoking about three weeks before this and
the first thing when I got over to the neighbor's house was ask for a
cigarette. I went over and told my mother and sister that they did all
they could but dad passed away. Of course, this upset all of us. Some
of the neighbors were over there. They saw the emergency vehicles and
came over to see what was going on. God love this one neighbor of
ours, Rosy Provost. I always called her Aunt Rosy. She was on the
heavy side and she came in. When she found out my father just died
she wrapped her arms around my mother. My mother was suffocating
and had to tell Rosy she couldn't breathe. Rosy meant well though. I
started smoking again. What they say is true whenever you quit and
start again it is worse. The first aid squad took my father to the hospital
because we all were upset. It would take a while for the funeral home to
come and pick my father up. My mother and I went up to the hospital
because we wanted to make sure the hospital did not have an autopsy
on him because the paramedics had a general idea what he died of. It

was just that my father had so many operations in his younger years we did not want him to be cut open any more. While we were at the hospital I went to see a friend of mine who was a patient there. It was my friend Bob. He had colon cancer. Within months he was also to die. When I got up to Bobs room his wife Joann was there. I hated to have to tell them the news of my father because they were going thru their own crisis at the time. I told them both that my father had just died. Of course, they could not believe it. No one could because he was ok to us. He was not sick that we knew of, he just finished a week at work. He did not have to take any time off so this was a shock to us all.

I called the funeral home that our family uses and within minutes the funeral director called me back. We set up a time to meet at the funeral home to go over the details which needed to be done.

Chapter 8

The Preparation
Prior to the
Funeral

All our family was always buried from Quigley Funeral home in Dover. The night my father died his body was taken to the hospital. The next day my family and I went over to the funeral home to make all the arraignments. My cousin Richard met us at the funeral home also which I deeply appreciated it. We all were in the office and I just needed a cigarette so Richard and I went out the back door for a smoke. I looked over near their garage and saw this stretcher with a blanket on it. At first it did not catch on to me but I thought for a minute. I looked at it and saw the workers going over to it and I said, "That is my father, isn't it?" They did not answer me. I asked again. Finally, they did answer me and said, "Yes, it is your father." I just freaked out and lost it. I put my cigarette out and went back into the office. Now came the time to pick out his coffin. We were looking for a simple wooden style coffin inexpensive. This was just another hard day. My mother brought down his cloths. All the arrangements are done. We are going to have two days of viewings, two times each day. Then on the third day will be the funeral. My mother and I wanted him to be buried from the United Methodist Church in Dover. My sister; however, did not think he should being he hasn't been in church for a long time.

Chapter 9

The Viewing

I did not realize how hard it is to do an old fashion viewing like we did for my father. Years later when it was time for my mothers' funeral we had only one viewing then the next day the funeral. The first day of my father's viewing we were shocked. We spoke to the funeral director and wanted for my father to be held in a certain room. This is because all our family has always been buried and laid out in this room. When we came in he was in another room. We spoke to the person on duty and he said there was nothing he could do because there is someone in the other room already. They were not going to switch my father. I made a big complaint. I called up the Quigley boys and told them what was going on. He told me that the person in that room was going tomorrow. They would switch my fathers' body and put him in the room we want. We came in and it was done. It was a hard two days. My father had a lot of people to come and pay their respects. I would go in and out in between smokes. I can remember the second night it was around 7:00pm, my mother and I was talking to a few friends. I never took my eyes off my father. I would always try to keep my eyes on him. Suddenly, I was looking at his arms and hands; it was like as though his one hand raised like he waved to me. It was not his physical hand it was like a third hand. It was like he was raising a spiritual part of his body. Well I flipped out. My Aunt Helen, God Love her, she has since passed on, came over to me. She took me down stairs to where they had a special room just for the family. We talked for a little while then we went back to the viewing. She had me come over to my father and touch him. I believe it was my father just waving to me in his own special way telling me he was ok. The next day was the funeral.

Chapter 10

The Funeral

We had just a few people at the funeral home then we went on to the church. There were a lot of people there. I held up ok. I told the person in charge at the funeral home I wanted to say something at the church. When it was the right time the minister called me up to the podium. My cousin Richard helped me up. I had so much to say but when it came time for me to speak I was lost for words. Basically, I just thanked everyone for all they did for us and spoke on how hard it has been the past few days. That was all. Then the song, "Amazing Grace." was sung. It came time to take my father out of the church. First was my father's coffin then my mother was supposed to follow. I got a little ahead of her because all my friends and co-workers were on the one side. I was greeting them till the funeral home director tried to stop me and put my mother in front. Well this got me mad. I made it all the way to the last pew. There was my good old friend Patty and her family. Her father was my fathers' supervisor. Well that was all I could take. I just broke down right there. I cried and cried. I got a hold of myself and moved on. We arrived at the cemetery. There was snow on the ground also it was very cold. The funeral was over and my father was laid to rest.

When we all got home it felt weird without my father and knowing he was not going to be coming back. We just took one day at a time. We knew we all had to move on. As time went on so did the grieving lifted from my heart. I will always miss you dad. You will always have a special place in heart and never be forgotten.

Chapter 11

The After Affect

Now comes the hard part, a time to grieve. I have had friends, neighbors, relatives die but never this close to home. It actually hit home. It felt as though the carpet was taken out of underneath me. I was close to my father, we both worked at the same factory. He and I worked in different departments on different shifts but we would still would see each other in between our shifts.

Well now it came time to come back to reality. There were just two questions that I had for him when he died. I believe in the afterlife so in my beliefs I felt he was still with me so in some way he could answer me. The two questions were: 1. Are you ok? I guess I am questioning if he made it to heaven or hell. In some form, I wanted him to answer me. Then question number 2 was what happened to you? I wanted to know what was the cause of my father's 'death? For those who believe will take this the same way I did. I had two dreams around this time and to me God gave me the answers that I was looking for. The one dream I had I saw my father leaning over and then I, in real life woke up in severe pain in the chest and the arm. I felt as though I was having a heart attack. Now I was fully awake. I was given the answer I had what happen to my father. I concluded that he had a major heart attack. The second dream I had of my father he was knocking at our door in our apartment in Florida. I said to him leave you are of the devil. He pleaded with me. Then I woke up. The next night I dreamt I was a work in the cafeteria and my father came up to me and pleaded with me to listen to him. So, we sat down and he said that he was fine. He did tell me he is in heaven now and will always be with me. He will be watching over me like a guardian angel. I believe my two questions was answered. I still miss him but it does give me comfort knowing what happened to him and that he made it to heaven.

Chapter 12

A Change to Come

It has been three weeks since my fathers' death. I am still having a hard time with it. I will be ok one minute then having to hide somewhere because I just could not hold back.

My mother made arrangements to see our friends in Florida for three weeks. My sister and I took her to the airport to see her off. I told her I will help take care of Teddy the family dog.

I was still on the midnight shift so I would stop by the house on my way into work. Teddy always looked forward seeing me. This one night I got out of my car and I looked up at my fathers' bedroom. I always had a habit of doing this. As usual his light was off like it should be. I took care of Teddy and whatever else I had to do at the house so I was ready to leave. I had to go to the bathroom before I left. Their bathroom was upstairs on the floor where my father's room was.

I went to the bathroom, when I was done I came out and looked at my father's bedroom. I could see his light was on, now I remember when I came in his light was off. This freaked me out, I ran down the stairs and out the door. I immediately looked up at my fathers' bedroom window and saw his light was off. I am thinking to myself what could this be? I do believe in the paranormal or the communication of the dead. Even today of me being a Christian I still believe in this. My conclusion of this my father is trying to communicate with me, just like he waved to me on that second night of his viewing at the funeral home. I spoke to my sister and she said that there were some strange occurrences she had witness to also.

I ended up keeping his car; my mother had no use of it. So, I sold my car and kept his at the time my fathers' car was in better shape. I took my father's death very hard. What helped me the most was just acting as though he was still with me. Today in my spiritual growth and what I have learned over the years as being a Christian I believe he is with me in spirit and watches over me. So, what I did when he first died and maybe for the first year after his death was whenever I would get sad and think him I would go for a ride. I would go in his car and go for a nice ride and I would just talk to him aloud as though he was sitting right next to me. So, if someone is reading this and grieving over the loss of a person or even an animal try what I did. Whenever you feel sad or that empty feeling inside of you and you feel that person is just not there start to talk to them as though they were. You know they just might be sitting right next to you. I think this was what got me through the toughest part of my fathers' death.

My mother came back to New Jersey saying she loved it down there and wanted to move to Florida. My sister and I just could not see it at first but after realizing how expensive it was in NJ and the difference down in Florida. We got together and decided to move after all to Florida.

Chapter 13

Suicidal

Once I moved to Florida all I knew was my friend Jimmy, his wife Donna, and his parents. Of Course, I also had my mother and sister. I left a lot of friends behind in New Jersey. I was so lonely and all that I have been threw I did not see too much of a bright future. I would start to think of different ways to commit suicide. The more I thought about it and came up with the different ways the scarier I was getting. The problem was though I just did not have the balls to pull that trigger, jump off that bridge or take that whole bottle of sleeping pills. I knew though I did not want to live any more so what can I do. I started to think about HIV and Aids how people die with this. What I did not realize or know that people can live for years with it. So, I became what I call passive suicidal. There were a lot of prostitutes in the town I moved in and the next town over. I would go out and pick one up and not use protection at all knowingly what I was doing. See therefore I say at that time I was passive suicidal. I thought that I would get HIV and Aids very easy by doing this eventually it would lead to my death. I did not know that it was so treatable and people lived for years with the disease. Well this just started out to be an occasional fling. The more I went out the more I wanted it. When my mania was at its peak I would go out around 7:00pm and not come home till 4:00 or 5:00am. This could go on for weeks on end. It does not mean that I was picking up someone all the time. I would just go out for the ride and see what girls were out. I remember a couple of occasions I did run into the police. I was cursing the next town over and saw a girl walking on the highway. I stopped and talked with her for a minute; boy you could tell either she was on crack or had some kind of disease. So, I made up an excuse and left. Meanwhile there was a police officer watching us and I did not even know it. Once I left he pulled over to her and talked to her for a minute then he came towards me. Well I knew I was in trouble, I did not have too much time because I had to pick up my mother at work. Anyway, he gets up to me and next thing you know the lights and siren goes on so I of course immediately pull over. He asks for my id and told me to get out of the car. Then he begins to question me about my conservation with the girl. I told him the truth that when I saw her I told her I was not interested and made an excuse then left. He did not believe me. The officer asks me, "Who would you like your car towed by?" I started to plead with him. I ended up making a deal with him, I will write an affidavit and be willing to go to court if necessary. He ended up being pretty cool. He said to me that I am a good-looking guy I should not need to be picking up prostitutes. Well he let me go and I was on my way to pick up my mother at work. I checked my wallet when I got down to her work I noticed the officer forgot to give me my license back. So, after I took my mother home I went back and picked it up. Did I learn my lesson? Did I stop picking up prostitutes? You most likely know what the answers were. That was no I did not. This just started to become a regular part of my life. I did not have a lot of money either. I got to know a couple of girls and when I first met them they very pretty; however, as time went by that changed. They just got into the drug scene and it brought them down quickly. I remember picking a girl up and not realizing it until she got into my car that she was pregnant. I just could not do anything with her. I apologized to her. She said that she was hungry so she asks if I would take her to McDonalds and pay for it. So, I said sure, I did not mine doing that.

Something I started to do to end my life ended up became an addiction to me. I went to a self-help group they had for a little while. Then I just got back right into it again. As you read on this addiction does not get any better it does just the opposite.

A friend of mine and I was going out one night to a hot night club. We were going down the strip and saw two girls looked like they could be hookers. We turned around and talked to them. My friend actually came right out with it "How much do you want to f—k? The way they were acting I got very suspicious; they did not act like real hookers. Then they were trying to get me. They were saying to me how about you. I just said to them I was all taped out. In other words, I did not have any money. Then they were trying to get my friend to buy dope from them. Once this happened I just knew they were undercover police. I said to my friend come on let's go. We were supposed to go around the block and meet them in the back. I told my friend what I thought and told him to just head back to our house and not to do what they said. So that is what we did. We started to head back to our town. Suddenly there was a police car behind us he put his lights and siren on. I knew we were in trouble. We pulled over of course and the usual is stay in your car, license registration and insurance card. Then more police cars came. After a few minutes, there was police all over. It seemed like the whole police force was there. They took my friend out of the car and were talking to him in the back of his car. I did not have to get out. I heard he was going to get arrested for solicitations to prostitution. When I heard this, I was startled. I got out of the car and told the police officer that we did not follow through with the actual thought. We went on our way the opposite of what the girls wanted us to do. Well I was told to wait until the Sergeant in charge of the case comes. He finally got at the scene. He comes over to me and I talk to him. He was very rude. He checked the tape of the whole incident and he not only told me my friend was being arrested but if I did not leave I will be arrested. They were trying to get something on me but they could not. So, I had to do a hard thing. He lived at home with his parents and my mother was over there this night. I had to call over there to tell them about this. It was so embarrassing. So, I drove his car home. Well needless to say did I learn from this? I still picked up the prostitutes but I always was on guard. I could always tell the difference between the police officers from the real ones.

Chapter 14

My Life Passed Me By

Well on one of those nights I went cursing something was going to happen that would change my life. I was traveling on a six-lane highway. There were three lanes on each side with a medium in the middle. I was going about 50 miles an hour and I was in the third lane, the fast lane. Something came across me and just told me to get into the middle lane. I tell you when I say this is no exaggeration and I speak 100% the truth. The moment I got into the middle lane I saw this bright light coming at me. I could not tell at first what it was. There was no time at all. The next thing I saw a car speeding pass me in the fast lane, the lane I just came from. He was heading in the opposite direction. I could not believe my eyes. Another car saw this in the other lane. The both of us turned around and went for a few miles to see if he caused an accident. Everything was ok, it was a miracle there was not any accidents because of him. If I did not move into the middle lane when I did we would have had a head on collision. I knew God was with me that night. It was not until a few years later when I was able to put this part of my life's puzzle together.

After a few days went by I was thinking what would have happen if there was an accident? It was in an area where there were no homes or businesses. It had been years but I use to be into C.B. Radio. I told my mother about the near miss and she agreed with me. So, I looked for the local C.B. Radio store. We went out there and told them what I wanted and they installed it in my car.

Well not knowing but this was going to be used for a lot of things. Before I was talking about being passive suicidal because of loneliness, God used this to combat my loneliness.

I would listen to the radio on my way home from work and I found this one channel with two guys on it. One guy's handle was "Hot Dog" and the other was "Believer." Their conservation would be so interesting. They would talk about the Bible and different things that are in it. Finally, one night I did get the "Balls" to cut into their conservation. I went by the handle "Keystone Cop". That was my old handle I had up in N.J... This was around the time I first started to come down with my illness. It had to be early 1990's. Gary "Believer" and I would get talking in the word of God, I loved it. Terry, "Hot Dog" was not a Christian, he was just the opposite and he would always try to change the subject. I remember Gary knew that I was sick. He led me to the sinner's prayer one night. I believed in God before and said the sinner's prayer but never publicly. Things were starting to change. I was not so lonely anymore. As far as picking up the girls sorry I still did it; but that did get better. I would not go out as much and when I did go out I would try to use protection. I did not expect to be perfect. Gary invited me to his church one Sunday. The only problem I had was everywhere I would go I always had to have a big mug of water to drink. I told him that he said that was no problem, bring it in with you. So, I decided to go. I met Gary and his family in the parking lot of the church. There were not a lot of people yet. We went up on the balcony and sat inside the church. What a place to be. It had a very nice view of the whole church. The time came for church to begin. Now you see everyone coming in. What seemed was not going to be a big crowd ended up being a full church. The praise team forms their circle around and each one holds one another's hand. You can since the Spirit of God is in this church. They broke apart from their prayer circle and immediately went into their place on stage with the opening song. This is truly the church my sole has been searching for. I felt like a changed person every Sunday when church was over. It would remind me of a nice spring Sunday back here in N.J. I can even remember when I was younger and going to church on Easter Sunday how beautiful of a day it would be. However, it was like this every Sunday down in Florida. I was not in the spot to get involved too much with the church. I needed to heard Gods word. I needed to be built up inch by inch, gradually. I did get involved into some of their functions. I remember the church hosted a coffee house down town on certain days of the week. I would volunteer and would go down some nights. I smoked at the time and boy would people question me about that. Occasionally I would get one of those people that would think we Christians need to live a perfect life. They would ask me, why do I smoke? and is it not a sin? But then I would answer to that all sins are forgiven. We all are sinners, every man, and women on the face of this earth. The only one true person who walked on this earth that carried none of His own sins but ours, that was Jesus.

By the way you are probably wondering the glorious name of this church. It was called "The Church of the Cross."

Well the more I went to church the more Gary and I would talk on the C.B. Radio about the Lord. This seemed to have brought a lot of people out of the wood work so called to say. Our C.B. family grew day by day and even as the weeks would go by the more it grew.

Well finally after talking to Terry "Hot Dog" for a while we finally met. He lived in a travel trailer in a mobile home park in town. Here I picture a guy with a round face, a Greg Brady Perm hair style type of look, maybe late 20's. I get at his place and first thing I hear is a dog. I do not remember if he told me he had a dog not. Oh yes, it is not just a normal mid-size nice type of dog that you would like to pet. Right off the bat the dog's name was Satin so i should think for a minute. Then when I came up to the dog I get some what intimidated. Satin is not a little toy terrier he turned out to be a Doberman pincer. He must have been at least 100 lbs., black with some brown in him. You do not want to get close to him. When I got over to his place, Terry had to carefully exit his trailer. Amazingly over a period of time I made a friend. I was the only one that Satin took to. Terry, let's just say had to go away for a while so I stayed at his place while he was gone to take care of the dog. The dog could not have been any better. I remember towards the end of Satins life he suddenly became very sick. Terry had to rush him to the emergency pet hospital. It was like 11:00pm and I went with Terry to help him. Satin was so sick that the doctor could do anything to him without sedation. Once the major treatments had to be done however; the doctor did sedate him. Amazingly Satin pulled through this. About 4 months later Terry was out with his hopeful girlfriend Teresa and his friend Satin eating lunch. Satin just lay down and died. It seems like he did not suffer, just as though he went to sleep.

Terry and I became good friends over the years while I lived down in Florida. He always loved the beaches. On the weekends, he would have cookouts for us on the ham radio or just anyone. One year we went down to Key West for four days or so. Another time we went to Orlando for a ham fest for an overnighter. He also would love to pick up the prostitutes. The only problem with Terry was he would not give them hardly any money at all. Usually he was a five-dollar date person. I used to give much more than that. Pending on who it was, how good looking she was could be twenty to thirty-dollar date.

First, I can remember meeting and adding to our family was Jeremy, his handle was, "The Transformer". Jeremy was 15 when I first met him. He also was like me when I first came into the family. Jeremy heard Gary and I talking and just broke in and the rest was history. We invited him to church with us one Sunday and he met us there with his uncle. Once his uncle met us he was ok. Then Jeremy was allowed to stay at church. As time went by I felt like I was being a big brother to him.

Another person came into our family was Herb. At the time, we first met him his father, George was about 70 + years old and dying from emphysema. His mother, Anna was a lot younger than his father. Hub's father was still able to drive yet but this was soon to come to a halt. I had the pleasure to have known George for about a year or so until he went home to be with the Lord. He was a very active member with AA for many years. I remember towards his last days he was just running out of oxygen as the days went by. The doctors put him in a nursing home for a few days so that Anna could get some rest. She called me up around 10:00am one morning and told me she was wanted at the nursing home. This did not sound good. I got over to her house as quick as I could. We got over to the nursing home. It seemed like it took forever. Anna went to the front desk and told the attendant who she was. Next, we saw a tall thin lady dressed in regular cloths approach Anna. She asks are you Mrs. Batchelder? Anna answers yes, the next thing out of the lady mouth was, "I am sorry; but your husband just passed away a little while ago. Anna was kind of expecting this when she got the call. It was still a shock. I know it was for me. I ask Anna and Herby if they wanted to come into the room and say a prayer. Neither one of them did. I checked with Anna to be sure she did not mind if I went in. So, I went into George's room, he was not covered up yet. I said a short prayer for him while I was with him. It was just as though he went to sleep. That is the way the nurse described his death. He ate breakfast with no problems at all. About ten minutes later he rung for the nurse and said he did not feel good, he was tired. Then that was all, he went backwards and went into his final sleep. Anna had a nice memorial service for George at Palma Sola Bay Baptist Church. Herb and his mother continued to be a part of our C.B. family.

Here is another important person that came into our family. Her name was Sherri and her handle was Giggles. I could talk to her till the wee hours of the morning. In fact, that is what we all use to do. We would carry on conservation till three or maybe even four o'clock in the morning. Of course, you would not catch any of us awake in the morning. Heck we would be lucky if we would be awake by twelve o'clock. Guess what, we all would be back at it again the next night. But back to Sherri when we first met her she was kind of withdrawn. She did not like to meet people. Her self-esteem was very poor. Sherri was on the heavy side; but she was a very nice person. Thru Jeremy going over to her house she eventually overcame this somewhat. She would come to church from time to time.

Bright Eyes, Doris was a friend of Sherri's. She would come on the radio also.

I remember there was for a while on Sundays we would fill one pew just with our C.B. family. There were others that came and went. Unfortunately, this also was to be for a season and we all moved on.

Before we did go our separate ways, Gary was an Amateur Radio Operator. He had his license to operate a ham radio. So, Gary talked Jeremy and me into going for our license also. It was not easy to do. We both went for the first test and that class license was Tech. I forgot how many questions there was to answer but we made it. This did not give us many areas to go. The next step was Tech Plus which entails another test. I thought the last test was hard but this one was to be the worst. It would be that of Morris Code. I think it took me about two months to study and get ready for it. It was a Saturday morning and I was put in a room all by myself. I finally finished and handed in my test. While I was waiting patiently the examiner checking the test came to me with a serious look. It looked like the type of bad news look. He came over to me with his hand and says "Congratulation" you passed.

To me that was a true miracle sent by God. You have no idea what Morris Code is like. I got my Call letter and they were "KE4AVC." Well to make a long story short it was worth it. I bought my first glorified C B which was also a ham radio. That was a Ranger RCI 2950. This radio you can get C.B. channels plus 10 meters which is in the ham frequency. I had a good time, the farthest I talked to was down under, Austria. I would talk all over the state and even all over the world. I am sorry to say but I did not renew my lenses when it was due.

All this time I was sick with bronchitis. Today I can see it as the beginning of depression. If there was nothing to do I would stay in bed. Especially when the C.B. family all fell apart I really went downhill. That was when I think I focus more on my illness. I was smoking a lot which I do not think it helped. I would try to quit from time to time. When Jeremy and I was Baptized at the Manatee Beach with our church I went under the water with my pack of cigarettes claiming I was never going to smoke again. Well that lasted for a day or two. I never gave up on quitting though. That is what people need to focus on. No matter what you are trying to give up you will be free from it just as long as you do not give up the notion that you will be free of your addiction.

I remember when Jeremy and I went to church he use to tell me not to sing too loud because I sang off key. Well one night I had a dream that I sang in a church choir and I sang on key. I told Jeremy about this and he remembers this. On his birthday, we had a little party for him and he told everyone a party about my dream. Funny thing is in 2005 my dream did come true. I joined our church choir in the Methodist Church.

We all ended up going on our own separate ways after some years that went by. I did enjoy our C.B. ministry and all of those that came across my path. I pray for those that are reading this by now are over their own dark days and are in their better times.

All this time I continued with my own illness. I thank God for putting all or the people at my side to help me get through the hard times. I suffered on a continuous basis.

I was not getting any better. I was trying to attack my illness with the medical perspective. I just did not know where to turn again. I figure that maybe I should try to see if it is psychological. So, it was on a Monday afternoon, I called up my Neurologist, Dr. McElveen's office. I spoke to his secretary and told her I was suicidal. Within 5 minutes Dr. McElveen calls me up and talked to me. He told me that he could admit me in the hospital and run some more test. I was in for about a week and did not feel any change. Dr. McElveen was ready to discharge me however I did not feel any better at all. I told this to Dr. McElveen and he suggested I see a psychiatrist while I was in the hospital. The psychiatrist came in my room and asked me some questions. She recommended for me to be transferred to the hospitals behavior wards. I was in there for about ten days. This was the best thing that happened to me. I was in group one day listening to other people's symptoms. After a while all the symptoms they were having I was having also. They called it panic attacks, anxiety attacks. Well this was the first time I could accept my illness as being psychological. I was put on some psych medications. They helped me somewhat but at least we were on the right road. This was just to be one of many hospitalizations. However at least I was able to come to terms of my

illness being psychological.

Chapter 15

The Move

We all moved to Florida in June of 88. I found a job in September
and started back to work. I guess things just piled up on me. I did have
a lot of pressure from work plus all that has gone on in the past. When I
first was hired my job was purchasing for the company. After a few
months, I was brought into the shipping department. My main job in
that department was manger in the department. I enjoyed it but with the
pressure it just took a toll on my health. It was a family operated
company. There were three brothers that owned the company. Their
father was the founder. I was doing well in the first six months to a
year. The one brother was basically in charge of the shipping
department. There was another person helping me in there as manager.
Well the one brother was giving us raises every month. I started there
at $7.00 per hour. Within six months I was making $9.50 per hour and
for Florida that was good money at the time. It was hard because I did
not know the product. So, we did make mistakes in there. Then the

other brother found out how much money I was making. This did not sit too well with him. Oh, the arguments the family would get into it was not funny. They all would go into their office and yell at each other. The other brother also had two sons which was a part of the business. Once all of this went down then the brother that oversaw me would take me out every day to the factory and would pass it on to me. He started to try to make me quit. I remember one day I went into the shipping room he said to me that there was going to be a layoff. I knew where he was going with this. Needless to say, I did not stay in the shipping room much longer. They realized that I was not going to quit so I was transferred to the factory part of the business. I was doing quality control work. That was the best thing they did to me. Then I started to learn more about the product that was they made. It was too late though, I already was starting to get sick from all the pressure. I was a smoker and with all going on in my life I started to smoke more. I was smoking at least two packs a day now. I would get so light headed and dizzy feeling. I went to the doctors and found nothing wrong. It finally took its toll and came to a head. I was on my way into work on

September 24, 1990 and it just felt like I was going to pass out. I think I was in work for just fifteen minutes and I felt like passing out. I said to my boss I had to leave that I did not feel good. I left and the more I was driving I decided to go to the hospital. The closer I got the worse I felt, finally I went by a gas station and I just could not drive any further. I pulled into the station and ask the attendant to call the ambulance. This was to be the beginning of a long, long mysterious illness. Even in my worst days I still smoked. However, I did stop drinking. I know my smoking habit did not help my illness. I finally had to quit my job. I just could not take it anymore. I must have been there for two to three years when I finally gave up the fight. I would never recommend for anyone to work for a family operated place. I decided to apply for Social Security Disability. From 1990 to 1993 I went to the medical doctors for my illness and had a lot of test done. At one point, I had a blood test done and it was determined that I had too much red blood cells. This is called polycythemia. I would have to go about every two weeks and have blood taken out of me. I was told by the doctor that smoking could be the cause of this. Did I quit smoking? Do you think this was beginning to scare me? The answer to both questions are NO.

I continued to smoke. In fact, I lit up a cigarette coming out of the

office where they took my blood from.

Chapter 16

The End of My Rope

I was at the end of my ROPE. I just could not take it anymore. I called my neurologist Dr. McElveen up and told his secretary that I was suicidal. The doctor called me right away and told me he will admit me into the hospital. He ran a lot of test and for the first time I saw a psychiatrist. The first time I saw her I was very intimidated. Dr. McElveen did find that I had arsenic in my system and he could not explain it. He ran another test and my levels were a lot lower. His conclusion was the test was an error. Back then they did not know about arsenic being from cigarettes so the test was accurate. Now today 2008 looking back and looking at the symptoms I had most of my problems was due to smoking too much. I was going to be discharge but I did not feel any better. I talked to the charge nurse that night and told her how I felt. She advised me to talk with my doctor so I did. I was transferred to their behavior ward for 10 days at which time I learned some about mental illness. Up until this point I refused to believe that my illness was psychological. I thought there was something medical wrong with me. Once I was in the behavior ward I went to the groups they had during the day. Well the patients would talk about their illness and symptoms. I could not believe that they were having the exact symptoms as I was having. All this time I thought I was having a stroke or a heart attack. I would think of all the illness out there and it just sounded like me. Finally, I came to accept that my problem was psychological. Once I came to accept my illness I then was on the road to wellness. I have to tell you it did not happen overnight. I was put on medication for depression and anxiety. Things started to get better. The reason I was feeling better in my opinion while I was in the behavior ward I would only go out for a cigarette four times a day, once after breakfast, lunch, supper and just before bed. We were only aloud two cigarettes each time so figure 4 times a day by 2 each time so I had a total of 8 cigarettes for the day. This was a big change from at least 2 packs I was smoking when I was home. I stopped looking in the direction of the medical field as far as my illness. Also, I was put on medications for my psychological symptoms. I think the cause of my illness was due to the stress I was under and also the

amount of cigarettes I was smoking.

Chapter 17

The Beginning of My Hospitalizations

This was to be the start of my revolving door policy I held at the psych hospitals in Florida. At one point, I did get a part time job as a security guard. Well as I mentioned the above policy I would work for a while and then get sick again and end up back in the hospital. My job was very good to me; they understood and accepted me when I went into the hospital. They always took me back when I was ready to come back to work.

I went to this one program. It was at a hospital in Tampa called Florida Mental Health Institute. The patients would live there for about two to three months. They had groups all day and some even in the evening. This place was like the others where we would be taken out for our smoke breaks. What the nurses or staff did not know we were smoking in our private bathrooms so I was getting more cigarettes than at this hospital then I would be normally. Unfortunately, I was at my worst during my stay there.

One Saturday I was tired and did not want to do anything. Well on Saturdays we all would have to clean the area where we would hold groups. I was told if I did not help clean I would lose my smoking privileges for that day. I just did not want to do anything. So, I got into an argument with one of the staff member that was on duty that day. He told me I could not go out to smoke. Ah what did I do? I just did not know why I did this but I was very sorry that I did it later on. I went back to my room and got a cigarette and my lighter. I came out and sat right in front of where the staff members would be. I thought I was being smart. I lit up the cigarette right in front of the staff member whom I just got into an argument with. Oh, did he not like it at all and was getting even madder with me. Of course, there was no smoking in the building at all so I was really pushing my luck. I was just doing it to be smart. Oh, did I get into trouble. He told me to put it out. I just smoked even more. Then he got more staff members and came over to me. He told me exactly what they were going to do. Like two staff members was going to take my hand the others were going to pick me up out of the chair and of course take the cigarette away from me. Now did this start me up even more. I fought with them as they were trying to get control of me. I would get to the point when I told them that I give up and they would start to release me but what did I do then. I would just start fighting them again. I really regret this today. I would have to say is respect those that want to help you. Have respect for all staff members where ever you go. I know that we all got bruises and markings on us from the refusal of them taking control over me.

I was really feeling bad while I was there. I was given a medication for anxiety and I would go for the medication at the nurse's desk. I would not take them right then. I would save them up. I slept my time here because I would take over the amount of the medication so I could sleep. I did this all the time. I just did not want to suffer so I figured I could sleep my time there. I regret doing this because they had a very good program.

Then my sister and I were not getting along good at all. She did not understand anything about mental illness and just thought I was just being lazy. I went home for the weekend and we got into a big fight. I got some of my heart medication and took it back with me to the program. I left the same day I got there. At a certain level, we could have our car there. I remember my counselor came in that Saturday morning because he really did not want me to drive because of the way I was feeling. No one could talk me out of it. Anyway, when I got back at the program I had a bottle of my heart medication. I went into my room and barricaded my room doors so no one could get in. They did a check of what everyone was doing every fifteen minutes. When they came to my room no one could enter. Well this alarmed all the staff. I told them what I had and I was going to take the pills. I told them I did not want to live at my home anymore because of sister. My counselor was great; he came in that night and tried to talk to me. Finally, after a while I came to an agreement. I came out of the room and gave them the bottle in return I was given an extra dose of my anxiety medication.

I have never caused any problems at any place I had to go except for there. That was when I started the procedure to get on disability. When

I found out how much I would get monthly I was happy. Finally, after several months being at the program I was discharge. I was almost sent to the state psych hospital. I told them that I did not want to live at home any more. The staff members talked to me about going there. They said that it is not too good there. People said that once you are in there it is hard to get out. Thank God, I changed my mind. Not too much longer I was discharged from the hospital. I regret sleeping the day away and not attending the groups. I know it would have really helped me if I went to the groups

My sister many years later will know what it is like because she herself experienced depression.

Chapter 18

Many Different Hospitalizations

During these five years we went through our problems with my

mother. She had a lot of health issues. I also had my own problems. I

suffered from major depression, at least that was what doctors

diagnosed me as. I would be what I called stable, being able to work

part time as a security guard then all my symptoms would come back to

me and bingo back to the hospital I would go. It was just like a

revolving door to me. I still believe the cause of the beginning of my

illness was due to my smoking. I would smoke at least two packs of

cigarettes a day if not more. One time I was in the hospital I had a test

done and it came out positive for arsenic poising. Today we know that

is one of the chemicals found it cigarettes. Smoking so many cigarettes

each day would build up my levels which would make me sick. Also,

you can get carbon monoxide poising from smoking too many

cigarettes. So, if we look back at the symptoms I had and the symptoms a person can get from both poisons I think I got sick from smoking too much. Then what would happen I would be in the hospital for a few weeks and I would smoke less. I would come out of the hospital, eventually I would start to smoke a lot and back to poisoning my system again

If you are a smoker work on giving it up. You also may end up like me if not worse. There are many programs out here now that anyone can get help. I pray that you quit.

Chapter 19

A Mothers'

Love

When we first got down to Florida we were eating at a buffet style restaurant. There was a sign-up Help Wanted so everyone was saying to me hey Bruce there is a job for you. Well the joke falls on my mother because we dared her to ask the manager if they had a job for her. She worked in a kitchen at a school for years. The manager was thinking of using her as a cashier but she hesitated at first. Then she ended up taking the job. She loved it and loved the customers.

Everything was going good for her but I forget what year it was when she started to come down with flu type of symptoms. As time went by she continued to get worse. Her medical doctor to me was a quack. He did not know what he was doing nor did the gastro doctor. At first her doctor, Dr. Martin thought that she could have cancer but why then did he not test her for it. Finally, she was so sick that she went to the emergency. I was sick myself at the time with server depression. Not knowing at the moment, she needed to have her gallbladder taken out and the doctor wanted to do it then. She said no to do it the next day. Well they were hoping that I would come over and talk her into doing the surgery that day. This was to be an illness that would eventually be the cause of her death. She was to last about five years. She also told the doctor how to do it. Boy what a patient. They do the surgery two different ways. The one way would be by using the lazier and the other would be the old fashion way, using the knife. Her doctor, Dr. Purifoy not knowing how bad her gallbladder was, did the lazier surgery. Her gallbladder was so inflamed that he accidentally nicked her bile duct. Usually it is the same day surgery but in my mother's case after the operation she did not feel good. They decided to keep her overnight. The next day her blood test shows that there was some type of infection in her system. On Saturday two days after the surgery Dr. Purifoy had to do an emergency exploratory surgery. I was in the hospital while the surgery was being done. Finally, after hours Dr. Purifoy came down to talk to me. The first thing he said out of his mouth was he nicked her bile duct when he did the surgery. So, it was his fault that this had happen. He explained the condition of her gallbladder before he operated on her and not realizing this. Her condition was critical, she may not make thru the weekend he warned me. Well this was to be the being of a long, long illness with her.

My mother was in the hospital this one time for a week or so. This one lady came into her room from Palma Sola Bay Baptist Church in Bradenton. Her name was Ellie and she was to be our Angel. She not only was a friend to my mother but she was there for my sister and me, during my hard days, my depression, back surgery and then my mother's death. Even today we keep in touch. The first day she met my mother we had a crisis. My mom was in the hospital for a while and my sister and I was in control of her monies, (Heaven Forbid). The day Ellie came in to meet my mother we had no phone service at the house. She was cussing up a storm. The phone bill did not get paid and they disconnected it. What do addicts do when they do not have money of their own? They go after other peoples' money.

74 of their own? They go after other peoples' money.

So, I dipped into my mother's checking out. (If my sister is reading this now I will most likely be hearing about it later). As I mention earlier about me picking up the prostitutes becoming an addiction I ran out of my own money. So, I ended up going into my mothers' money. Of course, I never said anything about it till now and yes, I did feel guilty. But getting back to poor Ellie meeting my mother on the first day going through this must have been hard. We ended up going to her church. My mother in fact was so scared of the water in which she was never baptized. Something just came over her and she was baptized at their church. It was a pure miracle. She would go when she could but the last few years of her life she did not seem to enjoy things too much like she did before.

We will have many dry runs of her funeral. She will come to amaze us many times of near death with her sugar level being up in 900 and something. She was not supposed to make it then but God was not ready to take her yet.

. We even got to the point where my mother was so bad the doctor prepared us for it. So, we called the funeral home up and made an appointment, thinking my mother was soon going to die. Well, my sister and I got over there and we did all the paper work, the planning. Then it came time to pick out the casket. You will not believe what we decided on. We saw this nice green metal coffin. My sister and I thought my mother could be buried with her green Stacy's' uniform. That is green and white plus the casket is green so it would all match. Well it ends up being funny. You may ask, how can this end up being funny? My mother continued to be in very guarded condition for days. She was unconscious most of the time. Amazingly this one day she just came out of it. Once she felt better my sister and I told her our plan with the green casket and her uniform. Well we knew she was alive. She said to us don't you dare bury me in my uniform in a green casket. Boy did she come alive. Things like this was to happen to her many times until she was to finally take her last breath with me at her bedside on July 28,1999.

Chapter 20

My Deliverance from Alcohol

I was drinking at the time a lot. I would go down to our swimming pool at the apartment complex at night. I would take a 12 pack every night. There was one time I remember when we had a scare of encephalitis. The mosquitoes were out in our area. We were told not to go out at night unless you had long pants on and long sleeve shirts. For the time being try to avoid going out if you can. Heck I did not care I did not listen to the warnings when I went down to the pool. I would also go swimming so I would only have shorts on. Later on, in my illness I went to a neurologist and he diagnosed me as being post encephalitis.

Well get back to my drinking. One night after the mosquito scare was over I was down at the pool again drinking. There was this lady and she was a Christian. She came over to talk to me. Well this was

the best thing that happens to me. I needed to quit drinking and we

talked about it. She talked to me about putting the full armor of God on

you every day when you first get up in the morning. I do not remember

her name but today I look at it and feel that just maybe she could have

been my Angel that God sent to me to help me quit drinking. She

prayed right there that night. She laid her hands on me. You may laugh

but I finished drinking that night it was to be my last. I woke up the

next day and felt no urge for a beer. Whatever beer I had left over from

the night before went down the drain. I would go to some AA meetings

sometimes. I would take my friend Jimmy with me. They had alcohol

free dance places on the weekends and AA meetings late on Saturday

night. Jimmy and I would go occasionally. Well I got through it, I

believe in the Power of Prayer. This was around 1991. I felt funny my

first New Year's Eve. We all went bowling. My friend Sharon Brooks

went with us thank God. I asked her "Can I have the champagne

toast?" I thought I could have just that. She said no. It was hard that night because New Year's Eve was always my time I guess you would say to tie on one. Today I have just as much fun being sober.

Chapter 21

My Symptoms

I continued to feel bad. Sometimes I would go to the hospital either by squad or I would take myself. This went on for three years. I thought my problem was medical. One day I just could not take it anymore. I was just staying in my room. Sometimes I felt like I was having a heart attack. I would get sever chest pains, numbness in my arm and all sort of symptoms. Then I would think I was having a stroke. As I just mention I would get numbness in my arms and it would go up into my neck. I would get weird feelings in my head. It felt like there was something going through my arteries in my brain. I just thought I was going to die. I would take my mother to the stores like Wal-Mart or the grocery store. If I had to go in with her I would have to use the electric handicap carts they have.

There were times where I would be in bed for months on end, coming out of my room at times. My legs would get so weak that it was like having to start to walk all over again. My mother and I would walk around the complex at night. Dr. McElveen also said that I could have something that has just started to come about. It is chronic-fatigue-immune-syndrome otherwise known as C.F.I.S... I found a counselor through my friend Sharon that deals with C.F.I.S... She was just in the next town over. I started to go and see her. I owed my psychiatrist money and got behind in payment so I started to slow down on seeing her. I was going away to see my friend in Indiana and I was out of one of my medications. This one medication you cannot just stop taking you must be weaned off it and she would not call any more in for me. I called my counselor and in return she calls my psychiatrist. She ended up calling me in a month of medication so I can have a chance to get another doctor. Well my counselor knew of a doctor up in Tampa that took care of patients that has C.F.I.S. so I went up there. He did a lot of test on me and did find something's out. There was a problem with my blood where I would have to go and have some blood taken out from me every other week. He did say that was due to my smoking. The doctor was about 1 ½ hour drive each way. Needless to say, when I got back to our house I would pass out. I got bad again one time with

81

this and just could not handle it so he put me in the hospital. He did some test and did some treatments on me. I had some type of liquids added into my blood system for a few days to see if that would help.

From 1993 to 2000 while I was living in Florida my hospital visits would range from two to four times a year. I would have to be very careful on how I regulated myself as to over doing it and on the other hand under doing it. Each time I was in the hospital was just like what we call a revolving door and that means someone goes out of the hospital and goes right back in. During my time in the hospital there were no groups or anything for one to do. The only thing we would have to look forward to do was to eat three times a day plus a snack at 8:00pm. It was just like we were in jail, eat, smoke and sleep. Then we would get four fresh air breaks for those that did not smoke and for those that did where given two cigarettes each time. I was still a smoker at the time. I would go into the hospital and I would start to feel somewhat better. Then I would get out and my symptoms would just come back again. I would go back into the hospital. I only had to be hospitalized twice when I moved back to New Jersey and that was in

2003 to 2004. Both of those two hospitalizations would be the answer to my prayers. There was a lot to do. There was a big gym, chapel, and many groups. There were many different activities to do also. We were not allowed to stay in our rooms during the day. This helped me tremendously.

Chapter 22

My Vacation

Well after my mother died my sister and I went through a lot and I just thought it would be good if I was to take a vacation. I went back to New Jersey for a week. I stayed with my friend Joann. It was the end of October and the leaves were changing. What a beautiful sight it was to see. It was so beautiful I realized I missed it so much that by the end of the week I had a mobile home picked out. I put a down payment on it then I decided to come back up in two weeks to make the final payment. It was a nice mobile home. There were two bedrooms in it. I called my friend Jimmy up to tell him that I was moving back to New Jersey. He just could not wait to tell my sister. By the time I called her up he beat me to it. She was all up set. I told her I would wait to move till after the holidays.

Middle of November came when Jimmy and I went to New Jersey. We were there for two weeks. I paid the mobile home off right away.

We only had to stay in a motel for one night. The next night we could sleep in the mobile home since it was mine now. I called up all the utilities like the phone, electric and cable to have them put in my name. The rest of our time we were up there Jimmy and I went around and visited some people we knew from years ago. We were kind of bringing back the old days. It was twelve years since I moved to Florida. It felt good coming back even though I was not moving back to my home town at least I would be close to it. My father was buried down in Dover also which I only lived about forty minutes from.

I got back to Florida, now came time for me to pack and put this mobile home up for a quick sale. I put signs on it and placed an ad in the local paper. I made a deal with one of the people who lived in the complex to handle all the dealing and she would get part of the money. It worked, not too long the trailer was sold. Now came time for the packing up. I decided I was going to use a little U-Haul trailer on the back of my car. This meant I could only bring a certain number of things. I went through all my stuff. I had a lot of just junk. It was like my parents Christmas ornaments which were so old. I either gave stuff to my neighbor or I just threw it out. It was a hard time for me because it was just a short time my mother had died and I was going thru all our family things. This was bringing up a lot of old memories.

My sister's job was not going too good. There were rumors going around there that they may be having a big cut back. We both talked and at that time I had some money. Now you must know me, money with me does not last too long. I told my sister if she wanted to move back to New Jersey I would help her out and she can pay me back when she got her money from her 401k. It was all decided she was going to move back to New Jersey. I was moving the middle of January 2000 and she was to follow April 2000.

Chapter 23

Back to New Jersey

Home Sweet Home

2000

I guess when someone dies in our family we pick up and move. Here I am back in New Jersey. I rented a U-Haul trailer and pulled it on the back of my car. Jimmy drove the car up. I did not have a lot of stuff. Figure I bought the other mobile home in November so I had time to get rid of any junk that I did not want. By now things was not going good for my sister at Winn-Dixie where she works at. She decided to move back also. We are not going to move her up till April. This way gives us all time to get things ready and for me to get settled. Jimmy and I got here January 17, 2000. It was the anniversary of my father's death. I was so glad to be home. The mental health agency that I was hooked up with in Florida made arrangements for me up here. You wouldn't believe it but the place was right next door to me. It could not have been any better or any closer. This ended up being a big blessing. I met with a counselor for the first two months then he recommended for me to go into their partial day care program. This turned out to be the best thing that happened to me. I went through many hospitalizations down in Florida and never felt like it helped me like this program did. I started out going to it five days a week. First thing in the morning there would be different work assignments the clients would attend. This would depend on what the client and their counselor would decide on. I got a job with their job crew. We would go to different places to clean such as; motor vehicle, Oil Company, fish hatchery and several more. I did this for a while and quit. I cannot remember why though.

Chapter 24

Quit Smoking Miracle

the Killer

Where do I begin to tell you the worst thing that I done to myself in my life? You may not realize it unless you your self have gone through the struggles, illness, and miseries in which this addiction brings on to us. The funny thing is we allow it to continue to put that nail in the coffin every single day of our life until it becomes our last. There are a very few that make it to an older age and remain symptom free. The rest of us start to suffer from the time we take our first puff till either the day we quit or we are finally put in that wooden box and that last nail is hammered in so we cannot get out. Oh, yes can you tell yet what is the worst thing in my life I did to myself? I pick up that first nail, that first cancer sticks, that my friends it was my first cigarette.

I saw this pamphlet at the program I was going to on how to quit smoking. I spoke to the counselor there that knew a little about the program. It was about forty-five minutes from me but I figure I would check it out. I called the number and spoke to this lady. She asked me some questions and I qualified being on a sliding scale. I felt good about the program. I met her husband Jim for the first time and I knew it was going to be a long road. I went to see Jim regularly once a week. There were some weeks I had to cancel because of my illness. Finally, I remember it was October 6, 2001 I felt very bad it was as though I was going to pass out, I also felt very nervous. I came into Jim's office and just could not go on that day. I told him how I felt. I was ready to quit. I told him that I am not going to smoke from that moment on, not the next day but that moment on. So, I threw out what ever cigarettes out that I had. I bought NiCoDerm CQ patch. At that time, I had to have a prescription for it. I used it differently because of my heavy addiction to nicotine. When it came time to put on a new patch I would cut it in half thus I was breaking down the dosage even more. I was doing this because I felt that I had a very bad addiction to nicotine. I only did this with my regular medical doctor's approval. Well I must say upon writing this February 2008 I am still a non-smoker. I tell people this short story. My mother God Bless, she went home to be with the Lord July 28, 1999. She got up there in Heaven and got on Gods back so much to help me quit smoking. He said to her, "Helen if I make your son to be a non-smoker will you stop nagging me?" She told Him, "Yes I will stop nagging you." Well from that time on I was a non-smoker. Thus, God is a Happy Camper once again.

Chapter 25

My Business Ideas

When I first came up here to New Jersey I had some money and the way I am I can never hold on to it. I bought a home business magazine and in it had an advertisement to buy jewelry at a wholesale price. I checked it out and bought about $3,000 worth of it. I went to the local flea market with my tables to try to sell it. I also had a catalog business I would promote. Boy did I have fun; the only problem I had was when I had to make the jewelry there on the spot I was too nervous my hands would shake so much trying to put the jewelry together. So, I still had some obstacles to overcome. I never did a killing but I think I would at least break even.

I also got into the pet breeding business. I raised hamsters, mice, guinea pigs and rabbits. Sounds like a lot of animals to breed in one mobile home. I would sell them to pet stores and to people. My favorite helper was there to give me a hand as usual. Yes, you guessed his name, Matthew. He seemed to have always loved anything I got into. I put an ad in the local paper to sell the animals along with a special kit. I would sell the animal with a cage, bedding, toys, and food at a special low price. I would be much lower than the stores would be. I loved doing this because I loved the animals.

Chapter 26

My First Paper Route

I was coming out of my home heading out on Rt. 57 and saw this guy by the motel hanging out. I said hi to him, and he said hi back. We started to talk for a while and finding out he just moved into one of the rooms in the motel. His name was Donald. This was to be the start of a long friendship. Donald wanted to start a paper route but the only problem was he had no transportation. So, he made me a deal he would give me gas money if I would take him. I agreed to it. Boy I did not know what I was getting myself into. We first started out with about 60 papers. Weeks went by and no money was coming in. The district manager kept on saying the check will be in a few days. That never came. Every two weeks was time for our customers to pay their bill. Some of them would send in their payment so we would never have to deal with them. Then others would pay us by check but they were writing the checks out to the paper company instead of Donald. Well I was beginning to realize he was not too good at the business aspect of the paper route. He eventually ended up turning it over to me. By now I got everything all straighten out. I had the customers write their checks out to me. So finally, I started to get paid. Don continues to help me most of the time. He eventually got bored of it and got into something else. By now my route is up to about two hundred papers a day, seven days a week. I am up early every morning, about 2:00am. I usually would get done by 6:00am – 7:00am at the latest.

Well I am continuing the partial day care program. I found another helper for the paper route. He ends up to the helper of helpers, again it was Mathew. I believe in Angles and God sends them to us in time of our need. He is the manager's grandson at our trailer park. His mother and grandfather passed away within a couple of years when I first moved up here.

Chapter 27

The Partial Day Program

The program I was going to was very helpful because I had a lot of issues I was holding inside. First thing when my mother died July 28, 1999 I got mad at God. I did not stop believing in him I still believed in Him, Jesus, and the whole concept of what is in the Bible. I was just angry at God. What happens to people when they get mad at another? Well with me I stop speaking to the person. So, in this case I did the same, I stopped speaking to God. I stopped my prayer time, going to church, and reading the Bible. I cut off all and any type of communication with God or anything to do with religion. I blamed the doctor who first operated on my mother for her death. I had a lot of issues that only by going to a place like this; the partial day care was I going to overcome them. There were groups such as grief and loss group, dealing with depression, self-esteem and more over the four years I attend there. It was amazing because on my paper route I ask my customers to save their aluminum cans, some did. The funny thing is I would be delivering the papers early in the morning. I would be so depressed that morning and by GOD what will I be collecting? Yes, a lot of cans. I would go into group that day and tell them about it. Even to this day I believe it was God reaching His hands out to me on those hard days. At the end of those mornings I would see the trunk of my car being full of cans. How could I not feel good? After I saw the pattern of this I knew that it was God trying to communicate with me. You have to be in the person's shoes that have experienced miracles first hand. There may be even ministers reading this right now that are saying this guy is bizarre, but trust me by GOD I know that I know. There have been times in my life I needed clothes and I had no money. Somehow someone came by and had clothes to give away. Thanks to the groups at the program and a dear friend of mine, Linda I came to terms and forgave God. We all need to learn forgiveness. If we do not forgive it just clogs our life up with hardships.

Chapter 28

My Spiritual Experience

Well if the talk about God communicating to me by giving me cans during my paper route makes you think I am "Off" wait till you here this.

I realized that God did no wrong it was just my mother's time to go. A friend of mine invited me to her church so I went. I ask for the pastor to come over to my house so I could talk to him. I told him how I was mad at God and it was thru him he lead me back into prayer. From that time on amazing and deep spiritual things has happen in my life. God tells me to tell people who are like Thomas the doubter "To have faith the size of a mustard seed" and believe. From this point on there may be some of you who may read this and just think I am "bizarre." Then there may be some of you who truly believe that these things really did happen and find these to have been deep spiritual happenings in my life.

I was going thru the shop-rite parking lot over in the next town. My friend Matthew was with me. Suddenly, I saw my mother, who passed away in July of 1999 go right pass me. I burst out in tears. Matthew tried to console me and told me it was ok he said go ahead and cry. Then this was the first time I put it all together. He said, "Mr. Smith I have been sent here to help you." Prior to this he would say to me how his name was in the Bible. He did not need to say no more. Then "Heaven" broke loose from that time on. I would be driving down the road and out of the clear blue a message would come to me. It would be in the form of a saying. I would immediately pull over and write it down. I made sure I went to church every Sunday. I enjoyed the music and the sermons. It felt good to have God back into my life. At that point in my life I felt I had the calling to get into the ministry. I made a lot of progress both in my psychical and mental health. I walked into church and people would say how it was a true miracle that happened in my life. I was on oxygen 24/7 for about two years and I was taken off it.

In June of 2003 I had a spiritual awaking. I felt as though God was talking to me and guiding me. Matthew helped me do the paper route with me this one morning. He did all the houses for me. I listen to the music and it was like God gave the music for that special time only because I lost it after that. I know it was God doing His works with me from that time on. I went home after that and it was time to clean myself from the inside out, like the bible tells us. I started to clean my house one room, one area at a time. Throwing anything that is garbage out. Boy was it pilling up out by my door. Matthew came over to the house and he tried to interrupt me. But it did not work. I would keep on saying to him "Divine Intervention." He finally left for a while. I had a problem with my sins and God knew it. He told me to go into the shower. Once I went in there He told me to pray and cleanse myself. This would be the way I can forgive myself and wash away any sins that I am having a problem with. Maybe if anyone else is having a problem forgiving themselves for their sins they can try this also. Now I was told hell is where you speak. So, to me it is here on earth. So, I stopped speaking. Matthew came back again, this time he had his grandmother call the police. The police came and I was just sitting in my chair. They would ask me questions and I would not respond. They saw all the stuff I threw out. The paramedics and my counselors were called out. I was just sitting in my chair and it seemed like my life went pass me. All my sins that I was holding in were coming out of me. You had to of been there in my seat to understand. I guess it was a form of scrooge, how he had the visits of the ghost. This was the same only I just had to sit in my chair and my life was going on right in front of my eyes. One of the police officers looked exactly like my paper route supervisor. The emergency squad members along with the advices of the paramedics decided to take me to the hospital. So now it was time to get me ready to go. They brought in a stair chair to get me to the ambulance. I got out side and one of the police officers tried to get me to talk again. I started to say a few words then I saw Matthew. I looked back at him with the type of look saying what am I supposed to do? I remember what he told me about hell is where we speak so in other words we live in hell. That was all I needed again, it shut me up. I remember the paramedic came into the ambulance and told me that he was going to be following us. He said that there may be times I may hear the siren and the lights will be on so do not get scared. Well we got down to the hospital in no time. I had all tests you could think have

101

done. God was still in contact to me. I believe I was being tested during this time. I went for a M.R.I. and when I got in there He told me to shake my head all over and fast when the test started. I had to think for a minute but I did what He told me to do. This was the same way with any other test I had done. I listen to God's commands; whatever He told me to do I did it. I remember hearing this nurse talking to a family describing the symptoms of a relative of theirs whom just died from having a CAT scan done with the contrast. This was exactly what had happened to my mother on the day of her death. I felt as though this was a message to me on what caused my mother's death. I had some feeling or something came over me to look over at the next room by me. All that is between us is a screen that you can pull away. So, I pulled it away and I saw this man sitting in a chair looking at the bed with no one in it. He saw me and pointed to the head of the bed. Then I closed the curtain for a minute. I open in up again and I was amazed on who I saw. It was my mother and that man was still sitting where he just was before. She looked at him and he looked at her and shook his head up and down like a yes. She looks over at me and with her lips says, "I love you". Here I am thinking that God wants me to go through the day she died again. So, I closed the curtain and I was expecting to see her again to see that final flat line once again. I reopen the curtain for the final time. This time there was no one in the room she was gone and so was the man. Questions we can ask, who was the man? Do you believe this happen? I believe and I know it had happened. I was there; I went through it and observed it. I have been told that people with mental health issues have that extra sense. I believe God has blessed me with many gifts and this is just one of them. You can believe what you want. Amazing things has happened.

Chapter 29

My Hospitalization

I remember the transfer from the emergency room to the state hospital. It was late at night. The hospital arranged to have an ambulance service to transport me there. The EMT put me on their stretcher and got a couple of blankets. Then I got covered up from head to toe. I have heard one tech say to the other "he is delivered now."

I got into the hospital and I was so scared. Someone told me at the self-help center I go to that the hospital was bad and she had a lot of problems there so I am going on what she said. The nurses brought me to the front desk and started to ask me questions. I am still not talking at all. They put me in the big bathroom where the front desk was and had me sit in a chair. They checked me all over. The staff was so pleasant to me. This small woman comes along; she must have been less than 5' tall. She tried to get me to talk and I still would not. She says ok "will you accept any medications we give me?" This time I shook my head yes. I guess they want me to sleep good because next thing you know the nurse is coming my way with a needle.

I think she was a Jamaican woman and she could not have been any nicer. Well she says Ok it is time for the shot. It is going to go in your behind. In it went and I did not even feel it. She said, "Ok Bruce common over here it is time for you to go to bed." I got into my room and they closed the door behind me. I thought they locked it. I was so scared I got on my hands and knees at my bedside just like I use to do when I was a kid. I prayed to God for his protection. Next thing I knew it was the next morning. Wakeup call was 6:00 Am., coffee and breakfast followed by smoke break was the highlight of the morning. I was so thankful that I quit smoking. This would now bring us up to 9:00am which now is medication time, then followed by community meeting which we would discuss anything that was going on and hear any complaints or comments. Different types of groups or church services would go in this time slot pending if people wanted to go as the saying goes "You can lead a Horse to water but you cannot make him drink it." Same case the groups are offered and for the people but they cannot be forced to attend. Also, here it would depend on what each person would do how quickly they would make any progress. Some people just stayed on the unit or in their room and those people are the ones that have been there for a long time. I remember one night I wanted to get out of there so bad I went to the exit doors which were locked. They were so secured that no one can get out. Well at least no one was supposed to. Somehow, I have no idea but I got the door open and once I did I went down the hall way with my arms open wide yelling, "Free at last, Free at last, Thank God I am Free at last." Well needless to say this was only for a very few minutes I was free at last. The staff heard me by now and realized I was wondering the hallways. They came out and took a hold of my arms. I felt as though I was a prisoner being caught from escaping. The staff was very good to me during this time I must say.

I stayed I guess you would call it in the catatonic stage for the first two days. Finally, my neighbor Paul brought Matthew to see me. I got into the visitation room and looked at him and in return he looked at me. I still did not know if it was ok to talk yet. I remember what he had said to me about hell is where you speak. I took that as to being hell is here on earth. I took up the belief also of hell being here on earth but that will be for another book. Any way I chose to open up finally and speak. So now everything started to get better. Eaman, Leann & Robert came in to see me. I also had the greatest surprise, my paper route manager and his manager came in to see me that made me feel good. I was only in the hospital this time for two weeks. When I was discharged I did not need the oxygen any longer. So, there was another miracle in my life.

Chapter 30

My Next Job

I started back to delivery papers right away. Matthew helped me as usual. He was always there when I needed him. During my paper route days, I had other helpers also from time to time. I do not want to forget them they were Glen, Louis, and Christy.

The self-help center needed a driver to pick up and take home their members so I took on a part time job with them. I dropped the paper route. Estella and Glen, two members from there came over to my house and ask me if I would consider the job. At that time, I was into my paper route so I was not ready to give up it. Not too much longer I took on the job. Their other driver Jim was sick. He had cancer so he just could not do like he used to. I took over the hours that he could not. It was not too much longer that Jim passed away. I took on the whole driving job. It still would be part time.

Chapter 31

My break down

November 2003

I was up and down in my moods. Thanksgiving was here and my sister came to my house for dinner. Before she came into the trailer we started to fight. I just could not take it any longer. I (what I call it to be politely) pored pancake syrup on her car window. We had the police come and they told her to leave. Well I ended up with a big fine for doing this. Next thing I was at the center and my friend Bobby came over, prior to this I was told he was spreading bad rumors about me. So, I told him to get out. He was not allowed to be in the center anyway. Let's just say it was a big argument. Finally, he left.

Well I wanted something and prayed to God for this to happen and it did not. So instead of getting mad at Him and doing like I did when my mother died I just thought I would go on a spiritual fast. I had been diagnosed with low blood sugar diabetes so it was important that I ate. I also was having a lot of problems with my back. On the third morning of my fast I was in terrible pain. I could not move or even get out of bed. I had Eamn and Leann call the rescue Squad for them to take me to the hospital. I got to the hospital and they were more concerned about my psychological symptoms then my actual psychical symptoms. I was in a lot of pain. I ended up getting admitted because of my mental issues. They asked me if I wanted to stay here in their hospital, not knowing what was going on I said no. The next thing I was on my way to the state hospital. I was in there back in June so I did not mind.

I was in the hospital for six weeks. They were very good to me. I saw a back doctor and he had me have a M.R.I. It did show a bulge disc. So, I had to have therapy twice a day. This started to help me about a week or so. Also, my medications where changed. I always attended any groups that I could or go to the chapel. It seemed like the longest six weeks that I went thru. I did a lot of writing while I was in this time. I was going at the nurses' desk for paper every five minutes. Finally, they got tired of me coming to them all the time. They ended up giving me a note book with paper in it. I did a lot of religious writings on what I thought about on many subjects or topics. I did not speak to my sister for about a year. I was in the hospital for Christmas and New Year's. They released me on January 14, 2004. I did not stay out of work too long. I went back to work in two weeks.

I progressed not only on my job but also in my illness. Driving for the center was a big help because it allowed me to go on different seminars. I got involved more than I thought I was going to. It became a part of my life and stopped being a job.

Chapter 32

The Calling

I have felt that I had the calling to become a minister at some point. I had some seminaries e-mail me and I believed that was God confirming my thought. I checked into one, I liked it. I took the information and catalog to Pastor Tim at our church to see if I could get any financial help. I gave it to him and the following week he talked to me. It turns out the church could not help. He did give me some advice which it took some time to sink in but it did. He told me that I should go over to the college and take up a few courses to see how I like it. Basically, the way I want to go about becoming a minister was going about it the easy way. So, I decided to follow Pastor Tim's' advice.

Chapter 33

Back to School Again

At some point, I decided to go to college. D.V.R.(Department of Vocational Rehabilitation) pays for schooling for those that are on disability so I went to them. Everything worked out and I was signed up for college and started my education. I took up psych courses for two reasons, the one was I want to become a minister at some point in my life. My first semesters I had to take up three refresher courses which I did not get credit for. They were Basic Math, Reading, and English which involved writing. Out of all three I ended up falling in love with English. I never knew how much I loved how to write. I have included in here my first pieces of work. I followed other semesters taking English courses. When I got sick back in November of 2003 I was put into Hagedorn Psychiatric Hospital and I wrote nonstop. You will see the writings in here also. I had felt as though God was inspiring me while I was in the hospital. It seems like I had so much to write that it just continues to flow minute from minute to minute, non-stop. I said to myself, "This could not be me, I am not a writer." Boy was I being given a lot of time. The other reason I wanted to take psych courses was I have been through so much with my own mental health that I want to learn. I wanted to get involved in the mental health field and learn as much as I can. Between driving for the self-help center and going to college I keep myself busy.

Chapter 34

The Birth of

Our Bipolar /Depression Group

September of 2006 I started a Bi-Polar / Depression Group. At first, I did not know how it was going to do. Today, two years later it is going good and we have anywhere from 10 to maybe 14 members attend it at a time this is on an average. We continue to have new people come in to join us. Some will stay with us; however, some did not. They may not be ready for a group yet. I urge anyone that has any form of mental illness to seek out a Self-Help group in your area. If there are no self-help group pertaining to your illness why not see how you can form one. It is not as hard as one may think. I have at the end of this book a series of organizations you can follow up on or you can e-mail me. I have enclosed my e-mail address. I will try to help anyone out the best I can.

Chapter 35

Better Future

Self Help Center

Another thing that I can say contributed to my recovery was our

self-help center. It is known as Better Future Self-Help Center. It is in

Washington, Warren County, New Jersey. I first went there for a visit

in 2001. I was not really into it yet. I remember one day two members

of the center, Estella, and Glen, I knew them from going to the partial

day program came over to my house. They asked if I could consider

being a driver for the center. They needed a driver. At the time, I was

delivering newspaper for the local paper and I was contented with that

so I turned the offer down. Not too much longer I cannot remember

what had happen with the newspaper route but I considered the drivers'

position for the center. I filled out an application and soon I was hired.

This was the best thing that happened to me. I would stay at the center

in between my runs. I started to get involved in the goings on at the

center. They would ask me to drive them to different seminars and conventions. At first when I took them places I was only doing it as a job. Soon I started to enjoy the different seminars we went on. I got something out of each one I went to. This was to be another item which helped me on that road to recovery. God knew where to put me. He put me at the very best places to learn, hands on learning experience. I even had the opportunity to go on a weekend convention. They went to Wildwood every summer for three days which I drove and had the opportunity to have a nice vacation also. I learned a lot over the years in which I was at the center. I saw a lot of people grow. However, I must tell the truth I saw just the opposite too. I have to thank a lot for everyone at the center from our Advisor, Managers, Facilitators', and all the members. Every one of them played a very important part of my recovery over the years. I also know that I played a role in my own recovery.

Chapter 36

My time as

Being a Facilitator

During the summer of 2005 there was an opening for a facilitator

which to me is an assistant manager. I put my application in and got

hired for that position. A facilitator was responsible for the center in

the evening. There were usually two facilitators on duty at a time. Our

detail responsibilities were to see the place was cleaned every night

should we do it or had someone do it for us. We normally tried to ask

for volunteers to do some chores. We would have to do the following:

- Wipe the dining room tables

- Mop and sweep the dining room floors

- Vacuum the living room

- Mop and sweep hallway

- Vacuum the library

- Take all the garbage out

- Clean bathrooms upstairs and down stairs

- Clean the porch for cigarettes

- Misc.

I did have my way with the members and others. If I did not agree with something I let the people know it. Maybe this was not the right way to go about things but I am working on it. I did like my job. I basically liked working with the people. As far as the cleaning details I think it was a waste of time. I think the members should be left alone. Perhaps some of the cleaning does not have to be done every day. Most of the members went to a partial day program from 9am to 3pm and when they get there they are tired. The last thing they want is to be bothered about cleaning. Is it the Facilitators job to do? I do not feel it is. If a facilitator is cleaning the time is being taken away where they could be assisting the members. The Facilitators' up most and foremost job should be made available for the members while they are there. I have heard of a member going to a facilitator and wanted to talk, the member was told that they were busy. They were in the mist of cleaning. These are where all the cleaning details should be written down and make a priority list. Then make a list for cleaning, most of it

119

can be done every other day. Thus, the members can enjoy themselves more at the club. Thus, the Facilitators' will have more time to spend with the members.   IT'S A MATTER OF OPIONION

Chapter 37

My New Job

I learned a lot while I was on that job. I traded hats in February 2008 when I gave up both my drivers and my facilitator's position. I took on the role a Peer Crisis Specialist. My duties were if there was a patient whom was in crisis at the hospital and they refused to stay in the hospital we would be called to go. Another person would go with me. Their title was a screener. They would interview the patient and determine if they needed to be in the hospital or not. If they determine the patient needed to be hospitalized then the patient had no choice. Now where my job comes in was to be there for support for the patient while waiting for the decision from the screener and doctor. I would sit and talk to them if they me wanted to. Also, if they needed anything providing the nurse in charge said ok I would get it for them. I remember years ago when I was in the emergency room in crisis I was all by myself and it was very lonely. So, I knew this job was very important. There were three of us as a peer crisis specialist. I have to tell you sometimes we would not go out for a while. I kept my self-busy writing my book or sometimes I would go into a room that was not in use and do a YouTube segment on mental illness. I even decided on a name to call it and it came to me just like everything else. I called it help4depression. I felt guilty because a lot of the time I was just doing my personal work. I liked it when I was asked to go to the hospital for a new patient. Finally, all the good things would come to a hard halt.

Chapter 38

The Accident

It was February 6, 2008, about 6:00 p.m... I was on my way to a speaking engagement for N.A.M.I. (National Alliance on Mental Illness) My partner Elena was with me. We both usually go together and speak to doctors, nurses, students, mental health providers, members of self-help centers and just the public. We talk about our experience of our illness. We were traveling on an interstate highway. It had six lanes, three going each way. At the time, it was dark but a clear night. I was in the middle lane going about 65 mph. There was a car in the fast lane going a little ahead of me. Suddenly, he got a blowout. His car got out of control. Everything happened so fast. He hit the left guard rail, and then his car went right across the highway, right in front of me. I thought for sure we were in for it. Well his car missed us. Then his car was heading for the right guard rail. Now I thought we were out of the woods because I figured his car would hit the guard rail and stop. Needless to say, I was wrong. He did hit the guard rail but bounced right off it. What do you think happened next? Yes, you guessed it. Suddenly his car hit my van's passenger fender and door. Damn I thought for sure I bought it this time. We came to a complete stop. I was just waiting for another car to come right around and hit us. Here it was rush hour. The van's air bag immediately deployed. Smoke suddenly filled the compartment. Elena and I both asked each other if we were ok I did not know how many times we asked. I went to open my door and it would not open, same way as the windows. Both the doors and windows were electric. Now my focus got off Elena and focus on myself. For a minute, I was beginning to question God because I came to the conclusion this was the end of my life here on earth. I prayed to Him and asked, "Is this it for me?" I was pounding on the windows with my hands. Cars was going by, even a tow truck went slowly past me and did not even stop. People were looking at me. Meanwhile smoke was still filling up. Boy did it smell. All this time seemed like an eternity. While all of this was going on somehow Elena crawled in the back of the van and got the door opened. I looked over to the passenger side and it was like an angel was there to

124

save me. It was her with the door open telling me to slide over and come out. Well I then knew God did have a purpose for me here yet. I got out of the van and Elena started to look for her cell phone. She left it back in the van. Then she saw other stuff of hers was there she left. The van was still smoking and I was afraid of fire so I was trying to keep her away from the van. I just could not keep her away, she just would not listen. Finally, it seemed like a long time a state trooper pulled up. I ran over to him and told him about Elena going back to the van. He went right over and told her to stay away from it. This time she listened. It just started to rain; we felt a few drops when the first aid truck pulled up. They came over to us and had the both of us go into their truck while we were waiting for the ambulance. Elena was having problems with her neck and shoulders. I had chest and abdominal pain. I think the chest pain was from the seat belt. It was not too long for the ambulance to come. They put me on a stretcher and had Elena sit on the bench inside the ambulance. Oh, what an ordeal this was going to be. We finally got to the emergency room. They put Elena in one room and me in another. The doctor came in to examine me. I was to have a series of test done. One of them was a CAT scan of my abdomen. We were there for quite a while. Fonda the other manager from the center came to pick us up. All my tests came out ok and Elena decided to stop treatment. She had to go to the bath room and they would not let her get off the stretcher but she could use the bed pan. Well she did not want to do this so she signed herself out. They gave me some good pain medication while I was there. When I left I kind of walked as though I was drunk. I even felt it. Yes, you bet I felt no pain then.

The following weekend the center had a conference to go on. It was about an hour and half away. To top it off I would have to get on a major highway right away. At first, I was thinking it was too soon for me to drive this long right now plus being back on a major highway. I was still hurting a lot from the accident. I have gone to this conference for about four years now. I just could not miss it. Well there was someone going along with us just in case I needed to take a break so this helped. I ended up driving the whole way down and back. I had a few flash backs of the accident but I got over it. I really did not enjoy the conference too much because I was still in a lot of pain and discomfort. I went to bed early each night so I would not have to suffer. Once I took my night time medications I would just fall asleep.

It was time to leave. Another conference came and went. I did go to some workshops over the weekend so it was worthwhile for me to go. Next thing I knew it I was home and that long drive was over.

Chapter 39

The Aftermath

A few weeks went past and I was in a lot of pain still in the same area. I decided to go to the emergency room. I gave the doctor the rundown of what happened and what was done for me at the other hospital. He had another cat scan done only this time it was done with contrast. I had to drink a liquid and wait for an hour and half then they did the test. The scan showed my gallbladder was slightly enlarged. Well the doctor said this was ok. Needless to say, months later and pain it turned out I had to have my gallbladder taken out. I did have gallstones. I still was having pain in my abdomen on the left lower side. The surgeon checked me out and found I had two hernias. The one was in the middle of my belly and the second was in the lower groin on my left side. He believed this was caused by the accident. When the accident happened my stomach and chest both hit the steering wheel hard. The doctor talked to me about surgery with all of this. I would have one hernia done one week, the other the following week then have my gallbladder out the week after that. This was to be scheduled starting Wednesday August 27, September 3 and last but least September 9 was to be the last of my surgeries.

Just before this I took my vacation. I already made reservations at a campground up in the Pocono's Pa. The weekend before the center had their yearly trip to Wild Wood and I always drove them down. So, this was another mini vacation for me. It was just from Friday to Sunday but I always look forward to it. I had to be cautious because I was still in a lot of pain. My vacation came and went too quick.

Chapter 40

The Operations

Now it was time for the first of my three surgeries. It was same day surgery. I think I was at the hospital about four hours or so. This operation was my lower left in the groin area. I was in moderate pain at first. I think I may have started doing things too soon. I went to church and did do some driving after four days or so. I did not know what I was in for with this operation. I was still recovering from this one and then came September 3, time for the hernia in my belly. This was same as the previous surgery, it was done same day. Now came time for the bigger one and that was to have my gallbladder out. I got into the surgery waiting area. I was all prepped just waiting for my doctor. He got there and came over to check me out. I like him, he is very considerate. He asked me how my lungs felt because I have COPD. Who else would know better if there was any congestion or not? I told him I felt fine. I was all wiped out physically by now from having the other operations I think. The doctor asked me if I wanted to go home after the operation if all was ok or stay overnight. With the way, I felt I told him I would rather stay overnight. I am glad I did because I had a bad night. I was very uncomfortable and in pain. There was one point during the night I was running a fever.

The next day I woke up and boy what a difference. If it was not for my first operation I would have felt great. I was ready to be discharged. My neighbor came to pick me up and bring me home.

Chapter 41

The Recovery

Well I recovered quickly from the two operations but the first one seemed to progressively get worse. This was the hernia on my left side near my groin. I had pain, numbness and it felt like needles and pins most of the time. It affected my private parts like my testicular and my penis. I felt where the incision was a bump on the inside of me. It moved as I squeezed it slightly. I went to the doctor for a checkup and he said everything looked good. About a week went by and I was still in pain. I was getting low on my pain medication so I called him up to see if I could get another prescription. I was able to talk to him, he asked me the date of the surgery and I told him. It had been a month now. My doctor said I should not be in this much pain now we will have to keep an eye on it. I have an appointment in two or three weeks but I did not think I could wait that long. I will see how it is the end of the week and see if I can change my appointment. I am just resting. The only thing I am doing is going to school for now which is one day a week for three hours. The rest of the time I am staying home running a very few chores. We will see what happens latter in the week.

Well today is Sunday Oct 12, I am having a lot more problems with my lower right side. Having discomfort and pain also I have been having diarrhea. I caught a cold right after I got out of the hospital. I got some over the counter medication which usually works if I catch it in the beginning. This time it did not. I went to my medical doctor the beginning of October. He gave me some antibiotics. The cough just continued to get worse and as that progressed so did the pain in my right side.

I was supposing to get my work men's comp check last Monday and it never came. I called about it and they keep telling me well it should come either the next day or so it was shipped the Friday before. I am beginning to think if it ever got shipped. We will so see.

Well I did get all my work man's comp checks. Finally, it came time I was supposed to go to work per the doctor however; I was still in a lot of pain and did not feel good. It was like a big problem me taking more time off from work by the doctor. It is like anymore today there is a certain amount of time to recover and that is it. Heck I just went thru three operations one after the other. Any way I took off just a few more weeks with the doctors' ok. This turned out to be the worst year of my life. I still was working as a Peer Crisis Specialist. I would go into work and just could not stay for my whole shift. There were some days I had to call off. I just was not able to do anything sometimes. It took a year for me to get over the one surgery. I did stop going to the surgeon because he said everything was ok. There just was not anything more that can be done just time and healing.

The following August I came down with bronchitis very bad. I went to the hospital and they admitted me. I was still wiped out from the past surgeries. Well I was in for a few days and came home. I decided that I just could not go on like this. One day feeling ok and go into work then another day where I felt so bad that I would have to come home. I had a talk with my supervisor and gave her two-week notice for me quit.

Chapter 42

My Enjoyment

I continued going to church all this time though. I even did a service on Sunday evenings each week. I enjoyed doing them. At night when I did these services I felt like I was being recharged. I felt relaxed and felt the Spirit around us. When I first started to do them, it was while I was still working as a Peer Crisis Specialist. I would prepare for each Sunday on my quiet days at work. It was a lot of work to prepare but it was great. I felt nervous in the beginning. I had to have the power point for the service to be perfect. After doing them for a while I got comfortable. Sometimes I would have a power point presentation other times we would just go with the flow. I knew what I wanted to talk about before the service. I had a few people attend but it was worth it. For the Bible does say, "When two or more are gathered He is at our mist."

When I first started at the church I had a meeting with the pastor. I was honest with him. I told him about my mental illness also about my sexuality. Oh, yes, I haven't told you that I am gay. Yea I know some people consider this to be a sin that you will not enter heaven, but you know the Bible does not just say about homosexuality it also says about eating meat, a whole lot of sins that are mentioned in the Old Testament which consequences are subject to death. I had a friend whom committed suicide. There is nothing in the Washington, Warren County area for the LBGT Christians. I wanted to start something for us. I had mentioned this to our pastor and he said to word it differently. We started a Bible study on Thursday afternoon. The pastor would run our study on different aspects of the world we live in today.

Everything was going good until the day it came out at bible study that I was gay. Regarding confidentiality I will go no further however I do have to say even in churches there is discrimination against one another.

Within a year I left the church. I had a chance to sing in another churches praise team but I would be just facing the same thing. Should it come out there also about my sexuality there would be people that may react the same way.

There is a church for LGBT Christians about 40 minutes away. It is called MCC, Metropolitan Community Church of Lehigh Valley. I was going there about five years ago for a while. My car broke down and just could not go there anymore. So, I think I may go back to it. I was there once recently and I know they wanted to start a small informal church for the LGBTS community. Perhaps this may be the answer to my prayer in the long run.

Time will tell.

Chapter 43

Relapse

It is the first week of December of 2008. What a week was I in stored for and was not prepared for. First, I had two reports due for my class. Tuesday was to be my last day also I had to take a final exam. So that was a pretty rough day. I wrote the first report back in October. My professor gave it back to me and said it needed some minor corrections. I gave it to Elena to do because she is good at wording things. Well I should have known it would be the very last minute I would have it back. It was the weekend before finals and I was supposed to call her on Friday to make the arrangements to pick it up. Her answering machine picked up. I call twice that day and had no answer. Then the weekend came the more nervous I became. All sorts of things went through my mind. Elena eventually was able to get my assignment to me.

Chapter 44

My College Paper

Bruce D. Smith

Psychology 183

The Battle of Psychotropic Medications

And

Weight Gain

As we find in any medications there are the good points in them and then there are the bad points. We need to look at the side effects of each new medication we are considering taking before we decide to take them. If you have any questions or comments write them down, feel free and take them to your next doctors' appointment. You want to be well educated on your illness. One part of any illness is the treatment and medications may be a part of it. Sometimes we may have to outweigh the side effects and take the medications anyway even though there are some side effects. If there are side effects ask your doctor how you can battle them. As we know weight gain is a very serious side effect on a lot of the psychotropic medications. There are ways to combat this. We will examine it as we go through this study.

Ok let us Get Down and Dirty, Lets Figure out What causes the Weight Gain:

- Antidepressants and Anti-psychotics were created to alter an area of the brain call the Hypothalamus Pituitary-Adrenal Axis (HPA).

    A. The HPA is a system of hormones and glands. The hormones within the HPA regulate serotonin.

    B. The psychotropic medications are made to increase the output of a hormone which is believed to lower the level in stress, depression, and symptoms which are all to be associated with mental disorders.

    C. The HPA system has a group of steroids hormones called Glucocorticoids which regulate carbohydrate, protein, and fat metabolism.

(1)   D. The HPA system needs to be in balance for the body to
function properly.

E. The Human brain will usually make up 2% of our overall

body mass; however, our brain will use up 50% of glucose

in the body. The brain depends on our glucose for energy.

F. Activity within this system makes the messages of "energy
of demand" and "energy on request."

G. The activation of the adrenal system inhibits glucose up take
by tissue, by inhibiting insulin release. This process produces insulin
resistance but increases hepatic glucose production.

H. With inadequate "energy on request," a condition called
neuroglycopenia (a shortage of glucose in the brain, also hypoglycemia.)

 Note: (1) A-H www.psychdrugtruth.com/weight.htm"If you want to
read the technical Data."

Patients more likely to choose a medication not to cause weight gain
than those which do. Even if the drug is either less effective or has bad

side effects. (Massachusetts General Hospital Clinical

Psychopharmacology Unit)

I have experience this personally from the beginning of taking

psychotropic medications back in 1990 to present. I was first put on

Wellbutrin and had very serious side effects which I took myself off

right away. I would not tell someone which is taking it today not to

take it not to because of the side effects which I had. Everyone is

different. What medication may work for one person may not work for

the next. I weighed about 225 when I first started out with my illness.

Then in 2003 I was put on some of the medications I call to be known

as the weight gainer drugs. There were three right off the top of my

head that I can think of which falls into this category. I can remember

back then I was not told about any of the side effects which could cause

me to gain weight. I know it is my responsibility to check on this;

however, since there is such a big problem with weight gain

medications the consumers or patients should be made aware of this.

This way the consumer will be able to plan just like the diabetic on a

healthy program to help decrease the possibility of any chance of gaining weight. We as consumers (patients) and the Doctors all need to work together. Once a consumer is first placed on any psychotropic medications the doctor/psychiatrist should go over the side effects with the consumer/patient about them. Then the doctor/psychiatrist should have places where the consumer/patient can go for further help to battle some of these side effects. Granted some of these side effects if a person may have may be normal however on the other had they may not be. Then the person should talk to their doctor and decided if they should or should not take that medication. On the other hand, we know that there are some side effects such as weight gain that effect a lot of people so we need to address this. This is the example of one where yes, the medication has a serious side effect and it needs to be addressed. But we need to learn how to battle it and overcome it. Such as any of the weigh gainer medications we should look at our diet and exercise. We need help and it is not easy.

First let me talk about my experience I had with the medications which causes weight gain. I first started out with my illness in 1990. I did not accept my illness as being psychological until 1993. That was when I was first put on the psychotropic medications. I was fortunate however I was not put on many medications which had many serious side effects. I weighed about 230 until the summer of 2003 when I went into Hagedorn Hospital. That was when I was put on some medications which had serious side effects. No one went over them with me. I gained weight rapidly. Next thing I knew it and I was close to 300 lbs. without exaggerating. There were three medications that I was put on which causes weight gain and one of them was Zyprexa.

I thought that I would discuss one of the medications which I was on and then let us see if we can figure out a healthy plan to combat this or if we decide to stop taking it. We always want to work with our doctors when we do anything regarding our medications. If they do not want to work with you then this doctor is not for you move on to another doctor.

I have chosen to look into Zyprexa and dig some information out

Facts about Zyprexa:

- It is an antipsychotic

- Changes the actions of the chemicals in the brain.

- It is used to treat Schizophrenia and Bipolar disorder

- Not used for conditions that are related to dementia

- May cause to have high blood sugar (hyperglycemia).

I have read the on-side effects of Zyprexa and basically the only one which can be worked on is weight gain. The others like with this one you would want to mention it with your doctor. Now we can look at some type of a plan to combat the weight gain. On the other hand, if you are happy with the results of the medication verses the side effects then leave well enough alone. No matter what you still want to mention it to your doctor.

Ways to combat the medication-induced weight gain.

1) Start Exercise

2) Do not over extend yourself on your exercise plan.

3) Educate yourself on your medications

4) Talk to your doctor

5) See what weight gaining medications you are on. Consider changing them to other medications which do not have the side effects of weight gain. But you and your doctor should decide this.

6) Proper diet- eat a healthy diet. Go over with your doctor or a nutritionist. In the beginning of your diet try to have some support to get you through the ruff days. This can be just as hard as trying to quit smoking or anything else.

7) Talk to your doctor and perhaps he or she may want to consider lowering the dosage of the weight gaining medications.

8) See if there are any Antidote Medications to help.

Here is a diet that on the Psychdrugtruth.com web site gave and some may just want to try. Check it out for a while and see if it helps.

There are 4 items which are needed to follow in the diet:

(1) Conjugated Linoleic Acid (CLA).

(2) Omega 3 Fish Oil.

(3) Vitamin E.

(4) Calcium/Magnesium.

All four works together as a team. They are to regulate the appetite and energy expenditure.

If you can try to make adjustments to your food habits. Try to eat the following ways:

(a) Eat only 3 meals a day with no snacks in between

(i) Start to do this by small steps though. Do not cut out snacks completely suddenly.

(b) Wait 5 hours before your next meal.

(c) Have your breakfast a high protein meal.

(d) Eat your dinner before 6 pm.

(e) Make sure dinner is your last meal. Do not eat anything else after dinner.

While dieting you want to be sure you are getting enough food; but on the other hand, also not over indulging. Following this type of a diet should not be too hard. You do not have to watch your calories just the amount of foods you are taking in. This will be an adjustment you will have to take. But it can be done.

Directions on taking the Supplements:

- Morning -Three Ultimate Omega 3 soft gels. 2 CLA soft gels. 1 200 I.U. vitamin e

- Noon   - Three Ultimate Omega 3 soft gels 2 CLA soft gels.

- Bedtime - One tablespoon of calcium/magnesium in water

  If you have any anxiety or insomnia do not use the

calcium/magnesium.

One place you might want to check out the price for these are at Vita Costwww.vitacost.com or you can call them at 1-800-381-0759.

Things to do along with the above:

Be sure to drink plenty of water. Water helps to remove the toxins out or your body. Exercise is very important not only does this contribute to help lose weight but it also helps work on our chemical balance in our brain. Weigh yourself once a week and same time measure your waist, chest, and hips. Try to have a partner to work with you on the diet and working out. Remember do not over whelm yourself. Do little tasks at first. Maybe just go for a short walk or if you have a tread mill at your means just use it for five minutes. If you mess up one day that's ok there is always tomorrow to pick back up where you left off. If you see that you lost one pound in one-week Congratulations! You do not want to lose too much at once. That one pound in a week will turn into 4 pounds at the end of the month.

So, we can see that the medications we take can cause serious side effects. Zyprexa like others we have found can cause weight gain in some people. However, all is not lost there are ways to battle this also. Try to follow the diet in which psychdrugtruth.com gave us and see what happens. I chose to stop taking Zyprexa a few years ago but I am on two other medications which are weight gainers so I still have a fight to battle.

My course I plan to take is to follow the diet I just mention above also switch one of my medications over to one which does not cause weight gain. This can be dangerous and you defiantly want to work with your doctor. I know if I start to have adverse side effects then I need to switch back to the original way. But we have more tools at our disposal now then we had in the 90's. We have new medications and technique.

From my insight over the past 15 years of experience I have had of first hand being on the patients' side of the topic I can see there needs to be some work and help from the doctors.

I do speaking engagements for NAMI from time to time and there was one time I did mention this topic. At the end, the doctor got up and made a comment on how the medications cause weight gain. He commented on how it is due to the lack of physical movement when one does get depressed. His opinion was geared towards being the patients doing and not the medication. Perhaps he is not willing to accept that there is work which needs to be done on their part just as the part of the patient. We need to unite and not to place blame. What I think needs to be done is for a study and present this issue to the psychic board and not to shift blame. WE NEED TO UNITE AND WORK TOGETHER. WE CAN FIND A SOLUTION FOR THE BENEFIT OF US. THANK YOU

Bruce Smith

Professor Deborah L. Lanza, M.A.

Social Psychology PSY 183 I

Tuesday March 4, 2008

Mid-Term

    1.   As I look for the definition of social psychology there is no one

given answer. I first take the definition right out of the book is "the

scientific study of the ways in which people's thoughts, feelings and

behaviors are influenced by the real or imagined presence of other

people." The other definition I want us to look at also right out of the

book is social influence "the effect that people have upon the beliefs or

behaviors of others. We can look at both definitions and they are

almost equal. I might want to ask in today's society why are there so

many hate crimes in the gay community? Just recently a 15-year-old

boy was shot and killed by another in California. My question in this

case is what prompted the other boy to go as far as actually killing the boy? Was it because he was gay? The other thing to note is the boy did just recently come out about his sexuality in class. However, I thought that there had been some progress in hate crimes against gays.

Another case we can look at is how does one person can bring a community to do anything they say or command. I reference this to the Jim Jones massive suicide ring. He convinced his entire congregation to take the poison to commit suicide knowingly. I would want to try to find out how can people get so brain washed to end their life because one person tells them to. We have to be so careful today of who we decide to follow.

How about right now? The election and Senator Obama, who is he? A lot of people suddenly are following him, even I. I was amazed when I booted up my computer today my Verizon page article headline read "Obama the new antichrist." I saw this and of course had to read it. There was not much to it. Depends on your Bible skills but could he be "the antichrist?" I will leave it at that. No, I am not off my rocker but in today's times anything can go. Sorry I am going into the religion aspect. But that is one form of how he used Senator Clintons negative campaign. He would change the negatives to be a positive. I will use just one example to show. Senator Obama believes we should go and meet with our enemies. Senator Clinton thinks just the opposite. I believe we should also. I believe Senator Obama is going to go all the way. He is going to be the next president. So, there are a few examples of how we can be influenced and to add it all up what to me is social psychology.

2. I can think of a group being like an organization in favor of doing something that may not be right. They tend to look at it and find a way to justify it to make it to be right and in that case if it was illegal now it will be legal to do.

I would look at a business with 10 employees selling stun-guns. In this case the stun-guns that the company are selling 75% deadly. I the owner of the company hold a meeting with the 10 employees and tell them that if these stun-guns was not used the people that used them would have been killed (I not knowing each case at all). I convinced all 10 employees to continue to sell the stun-guns. Next week I will try to sell them the Brooklyn Bridge.

3. Using the election this year I can come up with two examples and make distinguishes between them.

    A. An add with Senator Clinton she is giving all the facts of what she plans of doing should she be elected. She goes deeper and claims how she is going to attack each issue.

    B. Senator Obama had Caroline Kennedy along with her uncle, Senator Ted Kennedy to back him.

Sample A: Would be considered as central route strategy. It is giving all the facts that she can provide.

Sample B: Is using just certain way to persuade people.

4. Let us take one contextual factor at a time.

   A. Contrast Effects takes a product, item, subject or whatever you may have. We will take that example and will first make one not so good. Then they will create the real product, item, etc. and it will be the real product. With creating the poor or low-quality product the real product will look to be good or even to be the best over anyone that is available.

   B. Priming would be the factor of taking any giving situation and considering it. Then take out the main or prominent event in which are in the given situation.

   C. Decision framing is where we look at a potential problem and come up with the solution. When doing this we will look at the best way to solve it with the most gain there will be. We must look at all possibilities.

5. Heuristics are simple mental shortcuts which may be approximate rule or strategy for solving a problem.

A. The Representative Heuristic is when the reference is focus on the similarity of one object to another. This could infer the first object acts or seems to be like the second.

Example: We can look at the different stores we have today. There is Wal-Mart then there is Macy. Both stores are selling the same exact items, boxed exactly the same but sold at two different prices. Of course, Wal-Mart is selling their product for $10.00 and Macy's is selling their product for $15.00. If you knew this and would have to buy the item which store would you go to?

B. Availability Heuristic is when we make things to be easy thus bringing specific examples to mind.

Example: The other day I was at McDonalds and I order a large diet coke with no ice. When the lady gave me my order the coke had ice in it. I chose not to make a big deal of it and just take it like it was.

Chapter 45

Depression Sucks

What are my thoughts when I first start to go into my depression? I feel sad and lonely. I also start to feel anger inside of me. I do not know where that is coming from. The slightest thing I will project in a negative way. I have a big problem with projection. Projection is when you have an issue and you dwell on it. Then you come up with the solution in a negative way. This is one of my worst enemies. That can set me off into a low spell for a while until I confront the issue and almost 99.9% of the time it is always solved in a positive way. The way I projected it never came into play. So, you see all that negative energy I used for who knows how many days was all wasted. If you also have this problem the best way it should be handled I would see is in the following way. Let's say if John oversees something you are involved in and you have to get his ok. You take the project to him; however, it takes a while for him to check into it. All this time that is going by you can either project the worst or you can just be patient and consider that he will get to it when he can. So, patients are the best way to handle this. It is ok to check in with him to see if he has had time to check it out but do not worry. We know what the Bible tells us about worry. Trust in God. I have been ok with my bills. It is not that I do not have any, boy do I. I just trust in God that the money is going to come and the people I owe are going to either work with me or just have that big word I just mention and that is patients with me to pay the bill. Think positive someday my bills will be caught up.

Well I got off track a little as I was talking about me and depression. I really wished I did not have to shave or shower when I get like this. I just do not really care how I look and I would just rather stay indoors anyway. I have caught a real good cold with a cough. It came on me two weeks ago. I have been trying to medicate it with over the counter medication but it just is not doing it. I go to the medical doctor tomorrow. He should give me something for it. At least I have made progress. I do not get suicidal when I get like this anymore. I used to before sometimes, especially in the 90's when I lived down in Florida. That is when I would end up in the hospital. Now I get over whelmed with sadness and loneliness, so lonely that no one can realize it inside of me. I know Jesus is with me and is carrying me threw the sands when I need Him to. As I am writing this I am trying to look at what can help not only me but also you when the hard and bad days come in. I lived on the Gulf of Mexico in Florida for 12 years. I was about fifteen minutes from the beach. So, what might bring me up somewhat is just go back there again. I would think back to a day when I was sitting on the beach on a nice day or sitting by the pool at our apartment. We need to find the positive thing that helps us. For me to remember what helped me was write it down so I do not forget when I need it again. That is a hint to you, whatever helps keep a journal. I have found journaling is a very important tool in my life. It does not matter if I do it all the time but it does help if I keep up with it. One reason you can think journaling will help you it is just one form of venting. I can look back and see what issues I had and how I reacted to them. Then I want to see how I got either out of them or over them. This here alone can be a very useful tool.

I have found for some reason every year around this time of the year which is the beginning of October usually two things happen to me. The first is I come down with bronchitis and I get depressed. When I lived down in Florida I was able to isolate more so then living up here. That is where I was able to overcome my depression was when I moved back here to New Jersey. I have too many people and jobs that rely on me. I work part time as a Peer Crisis Specialist. That is my part time job which I work 20 hours a week. I am pretty involved in my church. I am a lay speaker for the United Methodist Church in Washington, NJ. The town I live in. Sunday is a busy day for me. I go to the 9:15 and 10:30 service. I am a head usher for the 10:30 service. I also have started a new service there at 7:00pm. During the week, I plan for the service. I am so fortunate to have these responsibilities that I have mentioned because they give me a reason to keep going.

Chapter 46

Sick Again

Saturday Oct 11, 2008

Well another day of being sick. I caught a good cold when I was in the hospital back in September. I went to my doctor last week and he gave me antibiotics but it does not seem to be helping. It feels like I could be getting worse. Every year around this time of the year I usually get sick. I am afraid it is affecting my muscles and my legs. My one hernia which I had operated on August 27 was bothering me a lot today. I just do not know what to do. The doctor says it has been such a time so it should be good by now. I just feel like everything may be catching up with me. I am going to see how I am feeling on Tuesday and if I am the same or worse I will call the doctor back up. I will ask him to recommend a good lung doctor for me to see. This just goes on and on. When I get like this it does not only affect me physically but also mentally. When I do not get any better I start to feel depressed. Then my depression continues to go in a downward slump.

January 2011 and still the symptoms of depression haunts me. Tonight, as I am writing this I am going through another cycle of depression. I try to fake it in front of people. I put on the face as though nothing is wrong, I will joke with the people to hide my true feelings. I start to feel as though people are against me. Do I really want to go on I ask myself? As I have mentioned in earlier chapters I fear too much of surviving my suicidal attempt. Why does life have to be like this? All I want to do is taking a pill to sedate me so I can forget the sad feelings I am holding inside of me. When I get like this all I want to do is hide inside of my safe place. For me my safe place is my home. My place is away from other buildings; fortunately, I live in a nice cottage. I know that I have mentioned of my faith in God. I think sometimes that is the only thing that keeps me alive. It is like the poem, "Foot Prints in the Sand." When I am at my worst I know that Jesus is carrying me. I know that He gives me the strength to carry on. And I am reminded of the progress I have made since I first started with my illness back in the early 90's.

Chapter 47

Flying what a rush

November 2, 2008

Flying what a rush

You are at the lane ready for take off

Getting ready for the rush

Now hearing the engines roaring like thunder in the sky

Your heart starts to beet with anticipation going to the sky

The plane moves as you are looking out of the window

Suddenly it feels as though there is nothing below

The reason is there is nothing below

You are now soring in God's country and what a sight

Now you see how small the world can be the higher you go

The pilot announces you are now 49,000 feet

Now you are above the clouds and you can imagine how close heaven

can be

You look above just to imagine what above can be

You see the ripples in the clouds

The wave in the clouds

Suddenly there is a break

Oh my God there is land

You may be Christian or any other type of faith

Or even some one that does not believe in a God

But when you been above

You must admit we all do have the same creator

And he is God

I thank Him for my rush

Chapter 48

What is bi-polar?

Bi-polar is known as manic depressive disorder years ago is an illness which the patient has extremes highs then extremes lows. The patient mood changes which alternates between manic episodes of abnormally high energy and it reverse to extreme lows of depression. People who are diagnosed with bi-polar may have it so severe that they may not be able to function at work, in family or social situations, or in relationships with others. This illness can become so severe where the person can become suicidal.

What causes Bi-polar disorder?

It has not been known yet what the exact cause of bipolar is. Research has found that it can run in families. It can also be affected by persons living environment or family situation. There is a chemical imbalance in the brain can be another cause.

A person having sleep deprivation or substance abuse, including caffeine can cause a manic episode. Initially stress may be a trigger in depression or mania. However, as the illness progresses, mood swings may not be caused by any specific event. Without treatment, your bipolar disorder may get worse, causing you to cycle more frequently between mania and depression.

What are the symptoms?

When a person develops bipolar they may have the following symptoms:

Mania may cause a person to:

- Be abnormally happy

- Be Energetic

- Be Irritable for a week or more

- Spend a lot of money

- Get involved in dangerous activities

- Be sleep deprived

- Feel extremely happy or very irritable

- Have a high opinion of them selves

- No need of sleep as usual

- Very talkative

- Be more active than usual

- Difficulty concentrating due to having too many thoughts at once (racing thoughts)

- Be easily distracted by sights and sounds.

- Act impulsively on reckless things, such as go on shopping sprees, drive recklessly, get into foolish business ventures, or have frequent, indiscriminate, or unsafe sex.

Depression may cause a person to:

- Feel sad or anxious for a significant time

- Feel hopeless or pessimistic

- Have slowed thoughts and speech due to low energy.

- Have difficulty concentrating remembering and making decisions

- Have changes in eating and sleeping habits leading to too much or too little eating sleeping

- Have decreased interest in usual activities including sex

- Having suicidal thoughts.

After the manic episode passes, the person may return to normal, but their mood may swing in the opposite direction of feelings of sadness, depression, and hopelessness. When they are depressed, they may have trouble concentrating, remembering, and making decisions; have changes in their eating and sleeping habits; and lose interest in things they once enjoyed.

A person's mood can change suddenly from mild to extreme. They may develop it gradually over several days or weeks. After a person has a manic episode they may return to normal or their mood may swing in the opposite direction and feel useless, hopeless, and extremely sad.

When the person feels depressed they may have trouble concentrating, remembering, and making decisions; having changes in their eating and sleeping habits. They lose interest in things they once enjoyed. Some people do become suicidal or harm themselves during episodes of depression. Some feel as if they cannot move, care, or think.

Bipolar disorder is a very complex illness. It is because there are many phases and symptoms. There is no one lab tests for the disorder. The doctor or therapist will ask the patient detail questions about what kind of symptoms they have had and how long it has lasted. In order to come up with the correct diagnose. a patient must have had a manic episode lasting a week (less if they had to be hospitalized). During the same time, the patient must have had three or more specific symptoms of mania such needing less sleep, being more talkative, behaving wildly or irresponsibly in activities that could have serious outcomes, or feeling as if your thought is racing.

Treatment:

Treatment is first done by medications to manage the manic episodes and periods depressions. The doctor may have to try several medications until finding the right combination to manage the symptoms long-term. The medications included are mood stabilizers along with antipsychotics. Antidepressants are used carefully for episodes of depression, because they cause some people to cycle into a manic phase.

Hospitalization may be needed while the person is in the extreme mode of the illness. This is to protect them from hurting themselves or others.

Along with medication another tool which will help in the treatment is counseling. A patient may want to find themselves a good counselor along with having a physicist. Also find a good self-help group for whatever their illness is. It is the best place for them to get support. For example, if they are bipolar have them look in their area to see where there is a bipolar group. If they cannot find one ask their doctor, or counselor. If they have a computer lookup bipolar, they will be amazed on what they can find on it.

Chapter 49

When is it time to call your Doctor?

By all means if you feel you need to and it is not on this list please call any way. This is only a guide line.

- Think of harming yourself or others

- Hearing voices

- Want to commit suicide or you know someone who has mentioned wanting to commit suicide

Warning signs of suicide include:

- Use of illegal drugs or drinking alcohol heavily

- Talking, writing, or drawing about death, including writing suicide notes, and speaking of items that can cause physical harm, such as pill, guns, or knives.

- Spending long periods of time alone

- Giving away possessions.

- Aggressive behavior or suddenly appearing calm

Be Alert

- Be on guard may be enough should your mood change.
  If your mood does not improve in two weeks or sooner
  call your doctor.

- If you have a friend or a loved one and he or she is
  experiencing a manic episode and is behaving
  irrationally have the person seek help.

Positives things to do

- Get counseling

- Go to some type of group therapy

- Talk about your problem

Chapter 50

Psychiatric Rehabilitation by the Consumer

The field of psychiatric rehabilitation as I found to be first started in the mid 1970's. Some of the principles and values could have been founded back more than 150 years. As we look at this we are looking today at recovery and wellness. We look at some various forms of ways to improve a person's mental health once one implements their treatment plan most times we see an improvement. The things you may see on one's treatment plan would be exercise, go out for fresh air, some type of meaningful activity, social support, connections to other people, friendships, spirituality. We look at any positive activity that the patient enjoyed doing in the past before their illness came on and suggested that they would put this into their daily program. One thing I have learned when I wanted to help someone was to find out the positive activity a person uses to do prior to the onset of one's' illness. This way perhaps the person may not be able to hesitate to implement it in their daily route. We want to make it easy for the person and not sent them up to fail. This thing I am mentioning are some of the things I have learned by going thru it myself either not by having it or by having it. We have noticed in time when one does this and get on the right combination of medication, counseling, group therapy the person has a real good chance of recovery. However, when one does recover they need to stay what I call in check. They need to continue taking their medications, need to continue seeing their counselor and maybe continue in any type of therapy they may be involved in. You may ask how long the person may have to do this. I have to perfectly honest with you I am answering this for me. I have been diagnosed with bipolar and my illness stared out in 1990 now it is 2008. I would say I have to stay in check for the rest of my life so I can continue having a good quality of life. I still have my highs and lows. However, with the tools I have my lows get taken care of quickly and I do not even need to be hospitalized. It was not until 2003 when I finally got placed on the right medications. Some people are fortunate and it does not take so long but for me it took from 1990 to 2003 for the doctors to find the right medications. So mental illness is different in some ways than other illnesses but in other ways it is not. Mental illness is just like diabetes. There is a chemical imbalance in the brain and pending on what type of mental illness you have how it is treated. So, there you have mental illness is a physical disease. We still have people looking at mental illness as being shameful or in a negative since.

I became interested in learning about mental illness because:

1. I wanted to learn about my own illness for me.

2. I wanted to learn about recovery for me

3. I wanted to learn about other mental illness to help other people

4. As I got well I wanted to learn more so I can become a professional in the mental health field and still help others as I move on in my life.

I think we are finding more today that a lot of people like me are being accepted into the field because of their life experience. As for myself I can tell you my history in short how I think I came to wellness. When I moved to New Jersey I was placed in a partial day program for a few years where I worked on some serious issues I had to deal with. Then in 2003 I was hired for our self-help center as a part-time van driver. I would pick up the members of the center in the afternoon and then take them home in the evening at closing. I started to go on different conferences because the managers would want to go and they did not have a driver so I was fortunate I was able to go. I was able to learn and this got me interested. Sometime in 2005 I was hired as a facilitator which to me is like an assistant manager for the center. I did both for a while driver/facilitator. Also in 2005, I started to go to college. I felt the calling to the ministry in the previous years so I knew I need to start college at some point. I decided I was going to go for my Associates degree in Psych & Rehabilitation. After I get that then I will go for my bachelors in religion. Well my time was not stopping at the center as a driver/facilitator. A new position opened in our agency as a peer crisis specialist and this was with their crisis department. I applied for it and got hired. It was only for 10 hours a week. There was special training and everything was going good. Well God was good to me, January came and I was asked by my supervisor with the crisis department if I would want to work 20 hours a week I did not think twice about it I said yes right away. This meant

I would have to leave my driver/facilitator job but that was getting old. So, I was looking forward to this. Well to sum this all up I took on the peer crisis specialist job. Also, I go around the state for an organization called N.A.M.I. I go with another person and we have a DVD to show. There are different segments of people's lives of mental illness. Then we talk about our experiences. This is called In Our Own Voice. So, I am active in the metal health field. I do short videos of my personal life history on YouTube. My YouTube name is brucedsmith1959 and you can find me on Facebook at Bruce D Smith.

When we first look at a person we would like to know what could have been the cause of the illness. Also, what are the strengths and weakness they had? We would like to also know what types of activities the patient enjoyed prior to the illness. We would also like to know the whole house hold history. All of these traits are important because they may become an important part of their treatment plan. Once a psychiatrist puts all of this together along with a reasonable time of observation hopefully they will be able to come up with the correct prognosis of the disease. This will give a direction of what type of medication to start off with along with the treatment. For me it took a long time as I mentioned to find the right combination of medication. Also, it was a combination of treatment that put me back on the road to wellness and recovery. It was group therapy, work, social exposure and learning about my own illness. The most important was my personal spirituality I could go to church even when I was in the hospital. I have to tell you my recovery did not happen overnight but it was a very good investment. It was like a new lease on life. I thank God for the Miracle He have given me every morning I wake up. I look back at my life before my illness hit me prior to 1990 to see what could have been the cause. Today we can tell the possibilities which could have caused my illness.

The following I can say could have contributed to my illness would be:

- Family
- My mother possibly had some type of mental illness
- My father died in 1988
- We moved to Florida

- I lost a lot of friends' due to the move

- I changed jobs due to the move

- I smoked cigarettes a lot 2 to 3 packs a day

- I was a heavy drinker

- At first, I had a good job however I ended up being under a lot of pressure.

- My mother came down with a serious illness

Chapter 51

How serious can mental health be?

Mental illness can just be as severe as person with a chronic physical illness. If it goes untreated a person may find themselves becoming suicidal. A lot of people with mental illness become so severe where the person becomes disabled to the extent they cannot work. I fought the illness for three years. I would be in and out of work. This just put more pressure on me because I would get flak from the people I worked for every time I was out. Finally, after three years going through this I could not take it any longer. I went in one morning and had my mind made up that was to be my last day. I did not even work that day. I just went in and told them I could not work there any longer and I was quitting. That was the last they saw of me. I was relieved; sometimes we have to make some major adjustments in our life for our recovery. That was when I decided to file for social security disability. I was fortunate I was living with my mother and sister.

Chapter 52

My Symptoms

I first started out with sever anxiety and panic attacks. They were so severe that I would rush myself to the hospital. The first time I went to the hospital was September 24, 1990. It felt like my legs were going to give out, they would feel very weak when my spell would hit me. Sometimes I would get chest pains with numbness in my arms and neck. Then I would feel dizzy, like I was going to pass out. I have to tell you this felt so real. Sometimes I felt like I was going to die. On September 24, 1990, I went into work and was there for 15 minutes, I just felt so bad. This was to be the first time I missed work for my illness. Well I left work I decided to go to the hospital just to get checked out. The more I drove to the hospital the more I worse I was feeling. It got to the point I could not breathe. I pulled over in a gas station and asked for them to call an ambulance. This was to be the beginning of a long, long illness. There was to be many times I would go to the hospital either I would drive myself or I would call for the ambulance to take me, most of the time I would call the ambulance. This was getting kind of old. I was getting no answer. Our family doctor however did say he thought it was depression and drinking. He advised me to go to AA and see if that helps. I took his advice and went for a while and quit drinking but I still had my problems.

As you read on I will talk more about my illness and where I was with it. I can say when I would feel sick I just did not see any hope at all. I never thought I would be doing the things I am doing today. I just want to say to those that are suffering from any type of mental illness do not give up there is hope. It may take time just have patience. I was in a dark tunnel seeing no light at the end of it. I am now not only out of that tunnel but I see the light.

Thank You God.

Chapter 53

Mental Illness vs Disability

Any form of mental illness can be so severe that it can disable a person for life. The sooner it is diagnosed and treated with the correct treatment plan whether it is with medication, counseling, or group therapy the less of a chance a person may be disabled for life. In my case I went out of work in 1993; however, I did take on part time jobs as a security guard in 1994. There was no stress or pressure on the locations I was at. I would be ok for a while and then I would have to be hospitalized again. My boss was very good; he understood and was ok with it. When I was released from the hospital I would take a week or two off then I would be put back on the schedule again and start to work. I only worked twenty hours a week. Even till this day I do not know if I can take on a full-time job. I work twenty hours a week at the peer crisis specialist job. I do other things to fill my day but I do it in my time. I can take breaks when I need to. I do not think I could work through a full eight-hour day, five day a week, day after day.

We also have to figure in our daily chores that have to be done as work. The person that does not have mental illness takes it for granted. They just put it into their daily schedule of things to do. We with mental illness have to figure out what type of day we are going to have if we can fit it into our day. I can say for myself I can only do so much in one day. I have made a lot of progress over the years although. My life before was for every hour and a half of activities I would have to rest for at least two to three hours.

Chapter 54

Stigma

Let me talk to you about stigma. I hope will have a better understanding on stigma after you read this. Stigma is all over the place when it comes to any form of mental illness. It is found even in a place that you will least expect it. Where do you think that may be? I will tell you; even today we still find it in our churches. I have witnessed it myself. I have the calling someday to enter the ministry. So, when I first went to this one church I wanted to meet with the pastor and talk to him. I wanted to know him and what the church had to offer. I knew the church already because I went there several years before; but there was another pastor back then. Well I told the pastor about my calling for the ministry and I wanted to be up front and honest with him. I told him I have diagnosed with bipolar the first thing out of his mouth was, "That would be a red flag right there." Well to me right there is several things, not only was I being stigmatized but I think it is also discrimination. There is a position a person can hold with having two years of service within the church. A person can be a licensed minister. This would-be part time only and that is what I was looking for. I was told by the previous pastor about this. I mentioned it to the new pastor about this. He said he would check into it for me. I knew I had no chance. Well our next meeting it did not go over good. He told me that in our district they are hiring only the students that are coming out of the seminary. Well we need to change things. There are ministers out there that do have some type of mental illnesses. They can hold the position. I did get to go for lay speaker's class and hold that position in my church. People out here in the world once they hear you have some type of mental illness become afraid of you more so than that of a person with diabetes or someone with any other type of physical illness. Now since I have been on the right medications and treatment and even before that I never was harmful to anyone or harmful to myself. A lot of people's stigma of mental illness comes in the lack of knowledge of the diseases. Perhaps if people would educate themselves more than that fear would subside.

Any person that is dealing with the public should go though some type of education in mental health. This would include police officers, the ministry, hospital staff, court staff there is more I know. Today we understand mental illness better and finding more people are coming into the wellness and recovery mode. So, we need to combat this stigma fear now with the public.

I have experienced by becoming a member and working at our self-help center a lot of people are coming there to get help. What I find comforting is when I have a person come in and seeing a change in them six months down the road this myself is a reward to me. I started the bipolar group at our self-help center in September 2006 and it does help people and it helps me too. I think there should be more self-help centers in the county and more monies put into them. Let them offer dinners to their members for free. Do more with the self-help centers? Let them be open in the day time. If the members are going to a partial day program and they are doing well then perhaps it is time for them to move on. Let them go to the self-help center during the day. This would be for free. It would cut cost down considerably. Then a self-help center could afford to offer meals and it would still be affordable

compare to the cost of one-person cost for the partial day program.

Chapter 55

The 2008 Election

Bruce Smith

2/26/08

PSY 183 I Social Psychology

When I first looked at this assignment I could not think of what I could do it on. It was not until towards the end of when it was due it came to me and it was right in front of my eyes. What do we have going on in our country right now? Yes, the presidential election   I can never remember an election being so cut throat like this one being. Maybe I just never paid so much attention to them before in the past. However, look at Al Gore and Bush election that was a circus. I guess we may find it if we look back at most of the elections in the past we may find the same.

When we first started out with all the candidates it was all over. I could not make up my mind who I was for. My mind was going with the attitude of not voting for a republican because of the way this past administration was. Then I thought I must look at the person themselves and make my decision from there. So, my quest was to become a little harder. I had to look at more possible candidates.

How does one choose a presidential candidate? There are many ways to determine who will be the best possible candidate. Of course, this will be your opinion and your decision another person may review the same information and think different. We all have our own beliefs and what we think the way things should be. One of the most important ways is by watching all the debates. While watching them I took notes so I can remember what each candidate was for. Not all candidates will be 100% for everything I am for either so I have to decide what is more important. Keep watching the news, read the newspapers, or listen to your friends, family, and your co-workers. The idea of the whole thing is to get as much information as a person can to decide.

I looked at all the possible candidates and right off the bat I did not like any of the republicans. So that narrowed my decision. By now it brings us down to just three people. Which this means it really brings it down for me to just two because I do not like the third. So, for me I have to decide either Hillary or Obama. At this time, I am more for Hillary. I do not like Obama because in his speeches he refers himself to President Kennedy which I do not like. Here we are asking what or how can we be influence and to what extent. I have a very good example here because when Caroline Kennedy a few weeks or so ago came out and indorsed Obama my decision made a change. Caroline, her self-referred Obama to her father. If I can remember correctly I do not remember her ever indorsing any candidate before. So, this is a strong example of how someone can be influence by someone else opinion.

This weekend was icing on the cake. I was watching CNN to see how the election was and could not believe what I saw. Hillary was going out of her mind. Apparently, Obama made comments about her and it made it to the press. What my thinking was about this situation how is she going to be with our enemies? Also, how would she be with future situations should they arise? We need someone calm, cool and collective. Not to be hot headed.

The two major ways I was influenced to make my decision on how I was going to vote this election are; a personal endorsement of Caroline Kennedy and the second was this weekend how she herself reacted on T.V.

Chapter 56

My Autobiography

From

1999 – 2003

My mother passed away on July 28, 1999. I stopped praying,

reading my Bible, and going to church. I must admit I felt guilty every

day that I did not do it. Later, I moved back to New Jersey and I met

this fifteen-year-old boy. His name was Matthew. He ended up being a

helper of helpers. He tried to tell me in his own special way that he was

an angel sent by God to help me. Well my friends with the experiences

and help he gave me I truly believe this even to this day. He has always

been such a big help to me. Oh yes of course we would get into our

arguments but we would always work thing out.

Well on June 13, 2003 God gave me a vision. He told me not to talk

until I tell you and the scripture says you must clean the inside first.

Well I took this literary; I started to physically clean the inside of my

house. Any statues I had that was broken I threw out. Matthew came over and tried to side track me. I would just say to him aloud, "Divine Intervention." This panic Matthew, he went home and told his grandmother. Next thing I knew it the place was full of police and first aiders. To this day I remember it all and I had all my wits about myself so call to say. I knew exactly what was going on around me and what I was doing. I listen to God and my decision was not to talk. I sat in a chair in my living room and it appeared my past was passing right by me. The wrongs that I have done were coming before me. It was kind of like my judgment day. There were different people coming in to see me, some of my Easter Seals counselors and different first aiders. Then it was time for me to go. The paramedics took me to the hospital for tests. I have to laugh because God was putting me through a test. He told me whatever test was to be done on me to mess it up on purpose. Make some type of movement so the test would not be good. So, during any type of x-rays I would have done I moved while the x-rays were being taken. Then finally the tests were done correctly all though. I do not know how strong your faith is but God was telling me to do all these things to put me through a test. I know I passed every test. After

I was done at the hospital I was then sent to the state hospital. I was so scared when I found this out. I had heard too many bad things about the hospital. I got into the hospital and they put me into a large bathroom right next to the nurses' desk to asses me. They had several aids and a nurse there. Finally, the doctor came. She tried to get me to talk and I still was listening to what God had told me not to talk until He gives me a sign. They wanted to give me medications by mouth and I refused, so then the needle came. The staff was all very good to me even though I was not cooperating. Well needless to say I was still going to get my dose of medication. Next thing I knew it the doctor came over with a needle and gave it to me. This made me very drossy. One of the staff was a very nice Jamaican lady. I can remember her to this day. For some reason, I put my trust in her right away. She told me to follow her and I did. I was taken to my room. The door was shut right behind me and boy did I get scared when this happened. I thought of all the bad things I was told that happened in there. I thought the door was locked behind me. Man, now I knew it was time to pray hard. This was the first time since I was a child I got down on my knees and prayed. I was at my bed side and never before did I feel comfort and safe. I knew that God was with me and I was in a safe place.

It was about my third day there and one of the aids came to me to tell me I had visitors. I felt strange. I went into the visitation room and I saw Matthew and Paul, my other neighbor. I did not know what to do. Should I speak? Is it time for me to talk yet? I looked at Matthew and he look at me with some confusion. I said to him is it ok to talk now? He said yes so, I was so relieved. I came out of my catatonic stage so call to say. Then I was back in the world of hell. Matthew told me before hell is where you speak. This was another reason I did not want to speak. I truly even today believe earth is our living hell. It is what we make of it. We can make heaven on earth also, depends on how we handle our life. However, when we die if we are born again we go to heaven and leave this earth for eternity. During this time God was ministering to me. I learned a lot during the twenty days I was in the hospital. I was released on June 30, 2003. I was on half the medicine I went in with and I was taken of the oxygen. When I came in to the hospital I was on oxygen twenty-four hours a day, seven days a week.

To me a lot of miracles had happen during these twenty days.

I was attending a church call, "The Chapel." From the first day, I entered those doors I felt the spirit of God.

Chapter 57

Day by Day

People may think that once we have overcome our mental illness
that we will never have a problem with it. Let me tell you I take one
day at a time. It is hard some days to even get out of bed and start my
day. The other day and even still yet today I am having problems just
doing the simplest of things. I enjoy using my computer whether it is
writing or even going on the internet. I have been having difficulties
just getting my computer off the table and onto my lap. What causes
this you may say? I do not have the answer but all I know is that I have
good days and then days I just wanted to stay in bed. Some people that
do not know anything about mental illness cannot understand this.
They think that we are lazy. They think that all we need to do is shake
it off and just get that computer on your lap. On some subjects, I am
very sensitive. I jump to conclusions too fast and not to wait and look
at the pluses and minus. I have had my experience with churches and
they still stigmatize mental illness. The one church I was attending for

about five years. At some point, I was sent a note stating that I was nominated to join their group for people with disabilities. Well I felt very good about this and even honored that I was nominated. I even went out as far as staying overnight at a local motel. I did not know how long it was going to take for me traveling nor did I know how late the meeting would be. I went to the meeting feeling good. Right in the beginning of the meeting we went around the room introducing ourselves. I told them who I was and mentioned that I was diagnosed with bipolar. Well I get the same thing as my pastor said when I first met with him. They said this brings up Red Flags. Then I heard two ladies that was there saying," Well I guess we have to include mental illness as part of our group." When she said this, it was not in a good way. Churches are very helpful with mental illness just as long as it does not involve the congregation. We would have our own separate meetings. When it came for mental health week every year I wanted to do a segment in our service. I wanted to include one of our members that also had some type of mental illness. Well my pastor first told me to watch my time I only had five minutes to do my presentation. I told him what I had planned. Then after that he told me to be very brief and do it in less than five minutes. Now we have this once a year and we cannot put aside a part of the service to recognize mental health week. It is in churches that we must pass on the education and what to do when they know of someone or they themselves are experiencing some form of mental illness.

I am going thru a little depression right now this very minute that all I want to do is lay down. I do not even want to stay out in the living room and watch T.V. along with being on the computer. I need to take a break and get back into it soon.

Well it is the next day after I wrote the above. I want to do so much yet it is hard to do the initial beginnings for the projects. I know it will go over good and it is needed but I just cannot put foot in front of each other. In other words, I just cannot even get past the first part of the project. I am trying to finish this book that you are reading right now. At times, I have put it up for months on end. If I spent 4 days out of the week it would have been done a long time ago. But let me tell you it is not all that bad. At least I do get out and go to work. I drive for a self-help-center so I have a good reason to get dressed and get out of my house. I also share with my groups what is going on with me. I had an appointment with the LPN that I see for medications. I told her what was going on with me. We looked at to see if there was any new medication in which I was put on. Well I have been sick with bronchitis and some of the medications can cause depression. So, I just had to go thru each day and pray for these hard days to pass.

At least it is not nearly as bad as it was in the past. Back in those days I would not even get out of bed. I had too many reasons for me to stay out of the bed. So, for you also who have this problem you will get over it. Best thing to do is talk to someone. If you have a doctor or a counselor, make an appointment to see them as soon as you can. Tell them all that is going on with you. It is important not to keep things inside of you. Even if you go to any type of group talk, do not hold things in. Holding things in can just cause you to blow up at some point. You can explode in many ways. I have mentioned in previous chapters what it all did to me.

Chapter 58

The Twelve Steps of Depressed Anonymous

1. We admitted that we were powerless over depression that our lives had become unmanageable.

2. Came to believe that a Power greater than ourselves could restore us to sanity.

3. Made a decision to turn our will and our lives over to the care of God, as we understood him.

4. Made a searching and fearless moral inventory of ourselves.

5. Admitted to God, to ourselves and to another human being the exact nature of our wrongs.

6. We are entirely ready to have God remove all these defects of character.

7. Humbly asked Him to remove our short comings.

8. Made a list of all persons we had harmed, and became willing to make amends to them all.

9. Made direct amends to such people wherever possible, except when to do so would injure them or others.

10. Continued to take a personal inventory and when we were wrong promptly admitted it.

11. Sought through prayer and meditation to improve our conscious contact with God as we understood Him, praying only for knowledge of His will for us and the power to carry it out.

12. Having had a spiritual awakening as the result of these steps,
    we tried to carry the message to other depressed persons and to
    practice principles in all our affairs.

                May God Bless You Who Reads This

Chapter 59

Where am I going?

My future, who knows, only God above knows. He tries to give us good opportunities and tries to give us what is best for us. But the final decision is ours. He gave us Free Will, the ability to make our own discussion. No matter how much He wants us to do that one thing if we decide we do not want to then we will not. Let us take a short look at the Prodigal Son. He was given lots and lots of money. Did he do what was wise? No, it was his decision to do what he wanted to do. But the amazing thing is when he came back home God open His arms again and welcomed him back. So, remember that no matter how many times we fail or do what we think God does not want us to do but do what we want to do God is still here for you and me.

May God Richly Bless You and Yours as He has Blessed me

Your Brother in Christ

Bruce D. Smith

My email address is bds07882@gmail.com.

www.ingramcontent.com/pod-product-compliance
Lightning Source LLC
Chambersburg PA
CBHW051457170526
45166CB00001B/281